DIABETES FREE

HOW TO TREAT THE ROOT CAUSE OF DIABETES IN AS LITTLE AS 11 DAYS

TABLE OF CONTENTS

MISSION

This book is dedicated to the activists and practitioners of natural medicine and natural healing around the world.

We cannot cure disease by blindly following the fabricated, toxic, and profit-driven therapies of the medical establishment. Since conventional treatments have failed to cure any diseases, we must create our own holistic therapies and alternative methods.

As such, all of my royalties on the sale of this book are being used to help fund the mission of educating people about natural health care and exposing corporate and government corruption.

Once you've healed yourself using these methods, I ask you to join my mission by sharing your positive experience with friends and family, so they know there is another path to vibrant health.

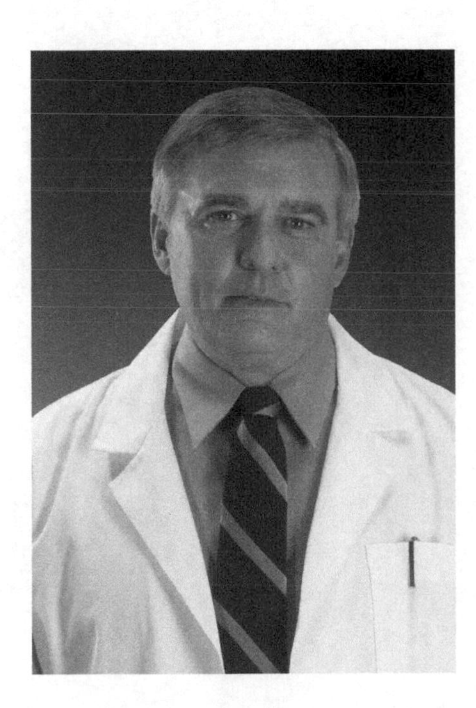

LEGAL DISCLAIMER

In this day and age, it is unbelievable to me that the world has come to this. It pains me that I must write a disclaimer at the beginning of this book.

Imagine – a person who is supposed to be allowed to express his opinions under the banner of "free speech" must still put a disclaimer as a preface to his words, thoughts, and opinions.

Lawyers are squashing the rights of people like me from freely expressing their ideas. So, with a figurative gun to my head, I write these words:

Before you read this book, you had better check with your medical doctor and anyone you feel is smarter than you and see if you can get permission to read what I have to say.

You must know that everything I say in this book is simply my opinion, and there are many people who violently disagree with my conclusions.

If you do anything, I recommend that without the supervision of a licensed medical doctor, you do so at your own risk. The publisher, author, distributors, and bookstores presenting this information do so for educational purposes only.

I am not making an attempt to prescribe any medical treatment, since under the laws of the United States, only a licensed medical doctor (MD) can do so.

How sad! So, this book is only my opinions, my thoughts, and my conclusions. Again, it is for educational purposes only, and you and only you are responsible if you choose to do anything based on what you read.

INTRODUCTION

Welcome to Diabetes Free. You've made a very smart choice in improving your health, and you're one step closer to reversing your diabetes.

As you probably already know, my name is David Pearson. I'm an independent medical researcher, specializing in Type 2 diabetes and insulin resistance.

And if you're tired of watching everything you eat, pricking your fingers, and taking injections or dangerous prescription drugs, this book is for you. The information you're about to learn will not only completely reverse your condition, it will also start repairing the damage done to your body as a result of having diabetes.

How can I be so confident? Well, I've spent over two decades researching diabetes and human health, and what I discovered changed my views forever.

It all started when someone in my family was diagnosed with Type 2 diabetes. Rita, who was like a mother to me, had a wonderful and vibrant life. That is until she went in for a routine checkup and found out she had diabetes.

In the beginning, it was no big deal. She did her best to avoid sugar and took a simple prescription drug to control her blood sugar levels. And it worked at first, but over the years, she got progressively worse. From one drug, she moved to two. And after a few years, she was taking a handful of medications to counteract all the side effects of the first few pills. And then, as she struggled to manage her blood sugar, she was finally put on insulin.

I could see firsthand the pain and suffering this caused her. I was the one who pricked her finger before each meal, and I could see the pain on her face as I did it. The worst was when I pricked her, and there wasn't enough blood for the meter or the meter just displayed an error message. I can still remember her face when I told her we had to do it again.

Then we had the insulin shots. She agonized over those. Maybe she was overly sensitive, but even though I was as careful as I could be, she yelped with each injection.

At the time, I didn't even realize there might be another way. We just followed the advice of her family doctor. But as the years went by, she got progressively worst, and I was at a loss as she faded away.

I was with her on her final night. She was unconscious, but I can still remember her squeezing my hand. I stayed until eight in the morning, when I finally went home to get some rest. I got a call at noon that she had passed, and I will never forget that day.

Something inside me ignited. I kept thinking to myself, "Could I have done something to save her? Is diabetes genetic? Is another family member next?" I had already lost a cousin to cancer a few years back.

And that's when I decided to learn more about diabetes and see if there was something I could do to make sure this never happened again. In the beginning, everything was new to me, and I wondered if I would ever make sense of what I was learning.

But as time went on (over 20 years now), everything started to come together, and I finally had a holistic understanding of human health that most doctors will never know. We'll get to why that is later in this book.

For now, I just want you to know that there's hundreds of pioneering researchers who are rising above traditional thinking and discovering breakthrough treatments for diabetes. Their work, along with mine, has come together to create this book.

I know I've finally found the natural treatment for diabetes. But don't take my word for it – everything you'll learn has been third-party tested and proven to work.

In fact, in clinical trials, this treatment worked 100% of the time.

So read this book carefully. Although this book isn't filled with medical jargon, the information it contains is powerful. I've discovered that I can reach more people with a straightforward, no-nonsense book that acts as a practical hands-on guide for what you should and should not do to reverse your diabetes. I'll leave the academic papers to solutions that don't work.

Some of what you'll read in this book is highly controversial. And it may even be violently attacked by Big Pharma, whose profits are being threatened. So, I ask you to read the whole book thoroughly before making a decision if this is for you.

Remember – what I'm asking of you isn't that radical at all when you understand the true cause of Type 2 diabetes. Unlike pharmaceutical drugs or surgery, this natural treatment doesn't have any of those dangerous side effects, so why not try it. As you'll soon learn, the real solution is a lot simpler than the medical industry has led you to believe. But before we get to that, let me take a moment to explain how this book is laid out.

In the first part of this book, I'll give you some alarming statistics about diabetes and how it's affecting our country. I'll share what's wrong with the current medical understanding and why pharmaceutical treatments will never work.

In Part 2, I'll open your eyes to the true cause of diabetes, discovered through fellow researchers and my 20 years of study.

In Part 3, we'll go over a 3-step plan to permanently reverse your diabetes in as little as a few weeks.

And finally, in the last part of the book, you'll find delicious recipes you and your family can enjoy while you're on this program.

I've risked my whole career on this! And I promise Diabetes Free is real, and it will change your life. It's time you discover how easy it is to become diabetes free. You have everything to gain and nothing to lose. So ... what are you waiting for? Let's get you started!

PART 1

DIABETES DECEPTION

CHAPTER 1

DIABETES: A GROWING PROBLEM

Diabetes is a growing problem in the world. In 2013, there were approximately 422 million people with diabetes worldwide (1) , and it's expected to rise to almost 600 million by 2035. Of those affected by this condition, 46% are between the ages of 40 – 59 years old. (2)

In the United States, the situation isn't much better. Approximately 30 million people have

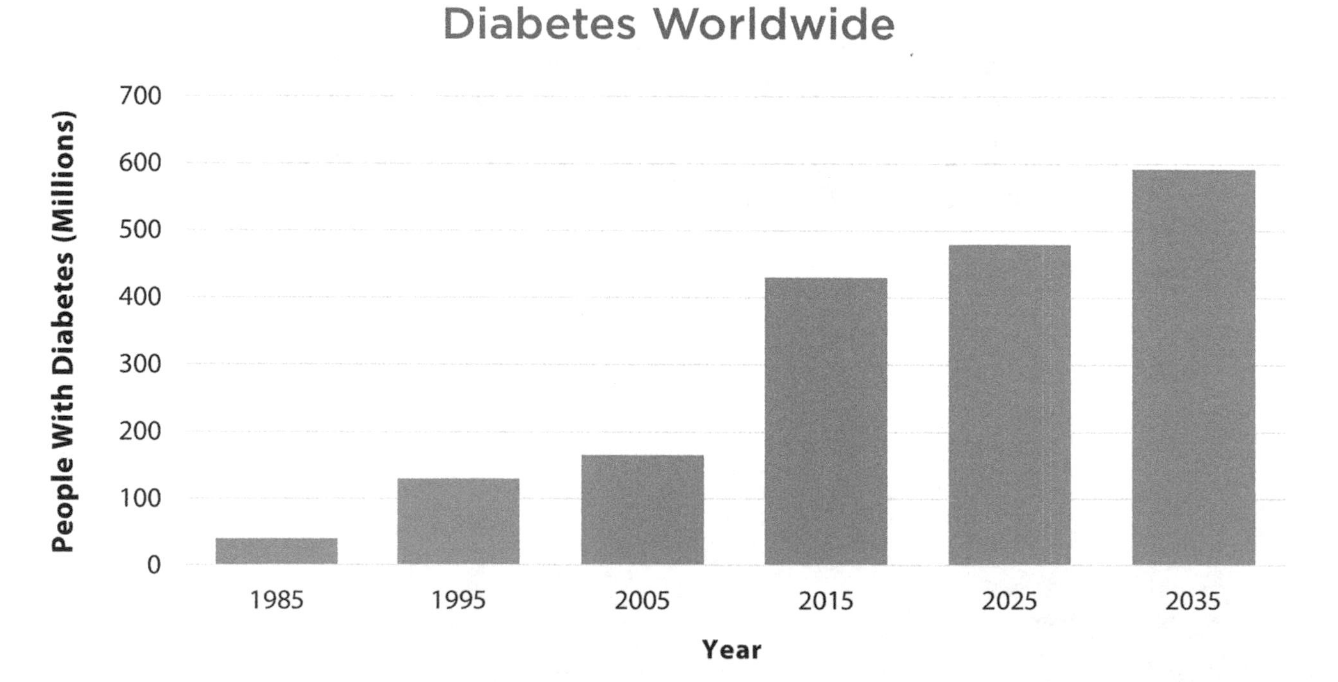

diabetes or about 1 in 10 Americans. And this number is rising drastically each and every year, especially in children.

What's scarier is that 1 in 4 people with diabetes don't even know it. (3) It's estimated that 86 million adults have pre-diabetes. Experts estimate that over 100 million Americans will be diabetic by 2050. That's diabetes in every family.

These are impressive numbers if you are a pharmaceutical company. But for everyone else, diabetes is a huge tax on health, happiness, and government resources.

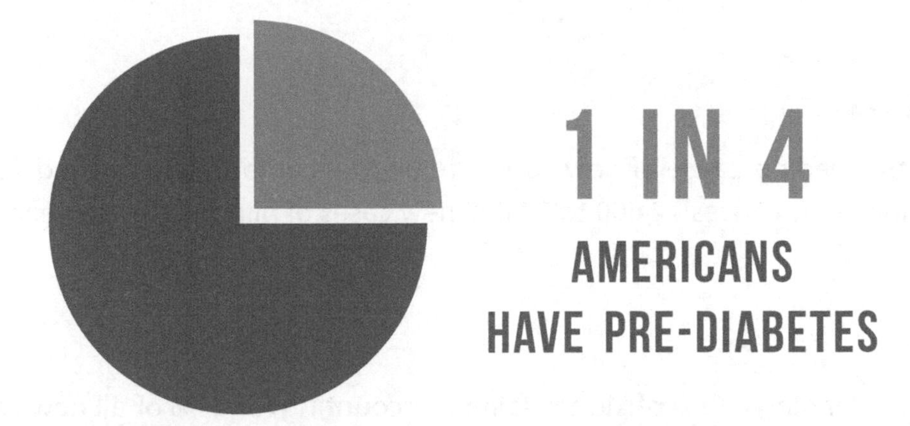

If you or someone you love is living with diabetes, you know how consuming this disease really is. It requires constant monitoring of blood glucose levels, medication, insulin injections, visits to physicians and hospitals, and more.

So why is it getting worse every year? And why hasn't the medical industry been able to control this epidemic?

We'll answer these questions in this chapter. Just remember – you'll never get a cure from the pharmaceutical companies, only ways to manage the disease. The only problem is that managing diabetes only leads to more complications.

Diabetes Complications

Having diabetes puts you at risk of a lot of other problems. That's why it's so important that you don't just manage diabetes but reverse it altogether. Current treatments don't regulate blood sugar very well. This leads to high glucose levels, and that's where the trouble begins. Over time, this causes all sorts of complications such as:

Heart Disease & Strokes

Heart disease and strokes account for about 65% of deaths in people with diabetes. The risks of heart disease and strokes are 2-4 times higher for diabetics than for adults without diabetes.

High Blood Pressure

About 73% of adults with diabetes have blood pressure greater than or equal to 130/80 mm Hg, or they have to use prescription medication for hypertension.

Blindness

Diabetes is the leading cause of new cases of blindness among adults aged 20 to 74 years. Diabetic retinopathy causes 12,000 to 24,000 new cases of blindness each year.

Kidney Disease

Diabetes is the leading cause of kidney failure, accounting for 44% of all new cases. In 2002, 153,730 diabetics were living on chronic dialysis or had a kidney transplant.

Nervous System Disease

About 60-70% of people with diabetes have mild to severe forms of nervous system damage. The results of such damage include impaired sensation or pain in the hands or feet and other nerve problems.

Amputations

More than 60% of non-traumatic lower limb amputations occurred among people with diabetes. In 2002, 82,000 amputations were performed due to diabetes.

Dental Disease

People with diabetes are twice as likely to have periodontal or gum disease. Almost ⅓ of all diabetics have severe periodontal disease resulting in infected and loose or lost teeth.

Complications of Pregnancy

Poorly controlled diabetes before conception and during the first trimester of pregnancy can cause major birth defects in 5-10% of pregnancies and spontaneous abortions in 15-20% of pregnancies.

Other Complications

Uncontrolled diabetes often leads to biochemical imbalances that can cause acute, life-threatening events such as diabetic ketoacidosis and comas. People with diabetes are more susceptible to illnesses and have worse prognoses.

The saddest part of all of this is that Type 2 diabetes is easily reversible. Unfortunately, this isn't a good business model for the pharmaceutical companies which stand to lose $55 billion a year. (4) Keep this in mind as we learn about how they diagnose diabetes.

Diagnosis Controversy

What I'm about to share is very controversial. But it's important to understand so you know what we are dealing with. Stay with me.

To help me explain, we first need to understand the difference between Type 1 and Type 2 diabetes.

Type 1 Diabetes – Your body **DOES NOT PRODUCE ENOUGH INSULIN.**

Type 2 Diabetes – Your body **PRODUCES TOO MUCH INSULIN.**

The difference between the two types of diabetes is very important, so pay attention.

When diabetes was first discovered, only patients who didn't have enough insulin received insulin injections. This is a true diabetic – what is referred to by the medical industry as a "Type 1". And this makes sense because they lack the insulin they need to metabolize sugar properly. This is easy to diagnose – just measure your insulin levels, and you get a clear diagnosis.

On the other hand, the diagnosis of Type 2 diabetes is not an exact science. It is a subjective art based on interpretation of vague symptoms, values, and subjective judgments. It is pseudo-science masquerading as an exact science. Don't be fooled by the standardized diabetes tests.

I believe the way they diagnose diabetes is wrong. Insulin deficiency should be the foundation of a diabetes diagnosis. Therefore, people who don't suffer from insulin deficiency **SHOULD NOT BE DIAGNOSED WITH DIABETES.**

Am I saying that you aren't actually diabetic? Sort of ... while symptoms you're experiencing are real and need to be treated, they're not the same thing as a true diabetic. And I think it's time they rename this condition to avoid confusion.

Here's my point – Type 2 diabetes isn't a disease. There's nothing wrong with your pancreas. There's nothing to be cured of. You just need to make some simple lifestyle changes, and your blood sugar will normalize on its own.

This is why Type 2 diabetes is so easy to reverse.

The medical industry doesn't want you to know this. The medical industry has lumped everything together to make this condition sound complicated and more dangerous. This sells more drugs and makes you feel hopeless to treat yourself.

Unfortunately, their incompetence leads to very real problems, especially in so-called "Type 2" diabetics.

Like I said before, Type 2 diabetics don't need extra insulin. In fact, they have too much! So when a Type 2 diabetic gets prescribed insulin shots, they end up having way too much insulin in their body. This is why Type 2 diabetics on insulin end up with the most severe complications.

If instead they treated Type 2 as you're going to learn in this book, Type 2 diabetes would vanish within a year.

Let's look at a few more diabetes myths.

Diabetes Myths

The medical industry will do anything to confuse you and prevent you from looking for solution on your own. Let's look at a few myths they use to stop you from trying alternative treatments.

Diabetes Is Caused By Genetics

FALSE – I want to make one thing clear. Diabetes is not caused by your genetics (5) . Genetics take thousands of years to change. People's genes have not changed in the last 30 years, but that's exactly how quickly the diabetes epidemic has come about. Also, in diabetes studies with twins, why are there cases where only one twin develops diabetes?

What's changed is our environment. We have lives with more stress, our food has gotten much worse, and we are all exposed to thousands of chemicals that have never even been tested for safety.

So the next time you hear someone on the news say the cause of a disease is genetics, remind yourself that most chronic diseases have only been around for the last century or so – nowhere near what it takes for genes to play a factor.

Sugar Causes Diabetes

FALSE – Diabetes is not caused by eating too much sugar. In fact, your body thrives on sugar; every cell in your body depends on it. The real answer is a little more complicated, and I'll show you exactly why sugar on its own is not the problem.

There Is No Cure for Type 2 Diabetes

FALSE – Diabetics are often told that they will have the disease for the rest of their lives. This is not true at all. Type 2 diabetes is 100% curable. There are thousands upon thousands of case studies showing it is very easy to reverse diabetes.

There Is No Cure for Type 1 Diabetes

Although this book mainly focuses on Type 2 diabetes, don't give up hope. If you or a loved one suffers from Type 1 diabetes, I encourage you to watch the documentary "SIMPLY RAW: Reverse Diabetes in 30 Days". You can find the DVD on Amazon or watch it on YouTube for free. Many people have reversed Type 1 diabetes as well.

The medical industry spreads these myths with the help of the mainstream media outlets such as CNN, Time Magazine, and others. In fact, Big Pharma drops over $5.4 billion on direct-to-consumer ads each and every year.

With all of this money exchanging hands, I don't think it's a stretch to say Big Pharma has some influence on the narrative of the daily news.

The truth is, the medical industry is completely clueless on the true cause of Type 2 diabetes.

The Current Theory

According to the medical industry, diabetes is a metabolism disorder.

In the case of Type 1, they say it is an autoimmune disease generally caused by genetics. Autoimmune basically means the body attacks itself. But why would your body attack itself? (We'll find out later.)

As for Type 2 (which is far more common), they say "insulin resistance" is the cause. They blame defects in your insulin receptors as the reason why your cells can't use your insulin.

If you look, you'll find volumes of research papers talking about these theories, but if you ask them what the underlining cause of not producing insulin or not using insulin correctly …

Their answer is "Cause Unknown".

Decades of research and hundreds of billions of dollars and their answer is "Cause Unknown". No wonder they have no cure – they don't even have a clue about what the true cause is.

The main problem is they've pigeonholed themselves into a box where only treatments that involve prescription drugs can be the answer. This is why they will never find the solution. I can't even begin to describe the pain, suffering, and death cause by their incompetence.

I don't want to spend too much time on conventional theories. If they were correct, there wouldn't be an epidemic of diabetes facing the world right now, and you wouldn't be reading this book.

In the next chapter, we'll learn more about conventional treatments and their dangers.

CHAPTER 2

THE BIG PHARMA CONSPIRACY

The Fake Search for the Cure

Just think about this for a second. How many thousands of dollars have you spent on doctors, prescription drugs, and insurance? After all that money, what results did you get? Are you beaming with health, or are you still sick?

Last year in the United States alone, $2.8 trillion was spent on health care – more than any other country spent. And yet, our rates of cancer, heart disease, diabetes, dementia, autism, and almost all diseases are some of the highest in the world. How could we be spending the most money on health care and research and still have the highest level of disease?

Diabetes medication has never even cured a single patient of diabetes.

In fact, the health and pharmaceutical industry hasn't really cured anything since the 1950s. Think about that. How many billions, even trillions, of dollars have gone into research for cures?

How many charities exist to collect donations to search for a cure? And after all this time and money, nothing has been cured in the last 65 years? How can that be? Don't believe me? Look it up. Try to find diseases that have been cured.

Yes, you go the doctors, and they tell you have "this" or "that". Just take some of this medicine, and you'll feel better. But do you ever really feel better?

Most pharmaceutical drugs don't even attempt to fix the root cause; they just try to manage the symptoms. It's like owning a car and seeing the engine repair light going on. And instead of repairing the engine, you just break the engine warning light. No more warning light, but how long will your car work until it breaks down?

And as you'll soon find out, not only do these drugs not work, they are riddled with dangerous side effects – including death! Just look at the warning label on most prescription drugs and ask yourself:

Is it worth all these risky side effects if it's not even treating the root cause?

The problem is they don't want you to be cured. Good customers are sick customers. That's the real reason there are no cures. Diabetes is a perfect business for them. You must buy medication over and over again … forever!

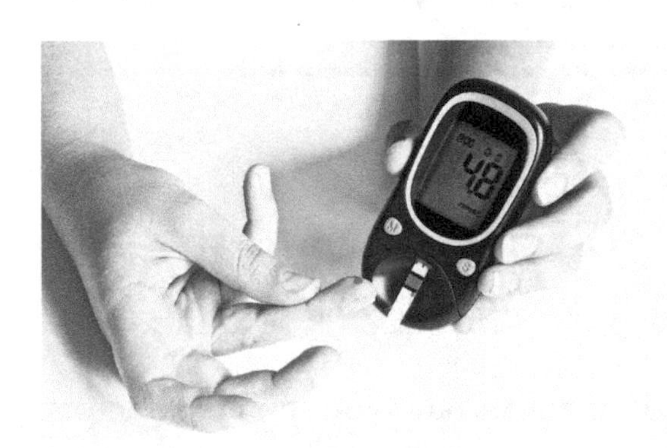

Big Pharma Profits

Think about this. **Diabetes alone is a $245-billion-dollar business and growing.** All those doctor visits, prescriptions, and insulin injections are making the drug companies a fortune.

The amount of money we spend on diabetes is continuously rising with no end in sight.

The major manufacturers of Inulin are Novo Nordisk, Sanofi-Aventis, and Eli Lilly. These three companies are making billions upon billions of dollars from insulin alone. Global insulin sales have increased 400% since the beginning of 2000, and they are growing exponentially. Insulin provides a majority of their sales, and they don't want these profits to stop. Just look at this quote from the former Editor-in-Chief of the New England Journal of Medicine:

"The combined profits for the ten drug companies in the Fortune 500 ($35.9 billion) were more than the profits for all the other 490 businesses put together ($33.7 billion) [in 2002]. Over the past two decades, the pharmaceutical industry has moved very far from its original high purpose of discovering and producing useful new drugs.

Now primarily a marketing machine to sell drugs of dubious benefit, this industry uses its wealth and power to co-opt every institution that might stand in its way including the US Congress, the FDA, academic medical centers, and the medical profession itself."

– DR. MARCIA ANGELL
(FORMER EDITOR-IN-CHIEF OF THE *NEW ENGLAND JOURNAL OF MEDICINE*)

Not only are these companies making a fortune, they also keep raising their prices. And why wouldn't they? They have no competition. Unlike most drugs that only have 10 years of patent protection, insulin has unlimited protection.

Yes, insulin is classified as a biologic drug which current law protects from generic versions. So don't expect discounts any time soon.

Corporate greed and corruption would all be worth it if these drugs actually worked. Unfortunately, not only do they not work, they cause a slew of other problems.

Toxic Drugs

Few people realize that prescription drugs have become a leading cause of death. **Drugs caused more than 2.2 million hospitalizations and 110,000 hospital-based deaths last year alone!**

Women, elderly people, and people with disabilities are least used in clinical trials, although they are the most affected.

Prescription drugs are now killing far more people than illegal drugs. And for the first time ever, more people were killed by prescription drugs than all motor vehicle accidents.

"Pharmageddon" is upon us. Pharmageddon is "the prospect of a world in which medicines produce more ill-health than health and when medical progress does more harm than good". And it is no longer a prospect, but fully upon us.

Diabetes Medications

The diabetes establishment uses several toxic pharmacological therapies in a deliberate but misguided attempt to control and suppress the symptoms and complications of diabetes. Anti-diabetes medication cannot cure or reverse chronic diabetes. These drugs are ineffective and can damage the kidneys, liver, and heart when used for long periods of time.

Diabetes drugs can even cause diabetes!

Some of these drugs are very dangerous. In 2007, an investigation found that Avandia increases the risk of heart attack, heart failure, and death.

This means that up to 100,000 deaths were potentially caused by this drug. (Drugs are supposed to help you – not shorten your life.) Just look at the scary side effects of these diabetes drugs:

CLASS OF DRUG: BIGUANIDES

Common Name: Metformin (Glucophage), Phenformin, Buformin

Side Effects: Lactic acidosis (Can lead to death), nauseas, headache, bloating, flu-like symptoms, immune depression, kidney damage, liver damage, upper respiratory infection, lung dysfunction, abnormal stools, chest discomfort, hypoglycemia, constipation, increased heart rate, muscle pain, nail disorders, increased sweating, light headedness, vitamin deficiency.

CLASS OF DRUG: SULFONYLUREAS

Common Name: Chlorpropamide (Diabinese), Acetohexamide (Dymelor), Glicazide (Glucotrol), Glimedpiride (Amaryl), Glipizide (Glucotrol), Glyburide (Micronase, Diabeta, Glynase), Tolbutamide (Orinase), Tolazamide (Tolinase)

Side Effects: Hypoglycemia, headaches, increased heartbeat, diarrhea, nausea, itching, vomiting, anemia, kidney damage, liver damage, heart problems, inflammation, immune depression, frequent infections, blood disorders, leucopenia, blurred vision, yellow skin, muscle pain, organ damage, obesity, joint pain, skin rash, autoimmune disorders.

CLASS OF DRUG: MEGLITINIDES

Common Name: Nateginide (Starlix), Repaglinide (Pradin), Mitiglinide

Side Effects: Flu-like symptoms, headache, back pain, drowsiness, joint infections, organ damage, coughing, immune depression, frequent infection, damage to pancreatic cells, hypoglycemia, blurred vision, seizures, coma, allergic reactions, autoimmune disorders.

CLASS OF DRUG: THIAZOLIDNEDIONES

Common Name: Pioglitazone (Actos), Rosiglitazone (Avandia), Troglitazone (Rezulin)

Side Effects: Congestive heart disease, hepatitis, edema, obesity, flu-like symptoms, headache, nausea, cold sweat, inflammation, bloating, obesity, muscle aches, blood disorders, liver damage, kidney damage, hypoglycemia, blurred vision, shaking, seizures, coma, heart failure.

CLASS OF DRUG: ALPHA-GLUCOSIDASE INHIBITORS

Common Name: Acarbose (Glucobay, Precose)

Side Effects: Flu-like symptoms, nausea, headache, inflammation, obesity, bloating, diarrhea, hyperglycemia, cold sweats, blurred vision, light headedness, shaking, seizures, coma, organ damage.

And these are just the documented side effects of these drugs. This list doesn't include rare symptoms that are completely unexplained. Insulin Therapy isn't much better.

Insulin (Hormone) Therapy

If none of the drugs listed above help control your blood sugar levels, the next thing doctors try is insulin injections.

If you're a Type 1 diabetic, insulin makes sense. But as a Type 2 diabetic, insulin only leads to more problems.

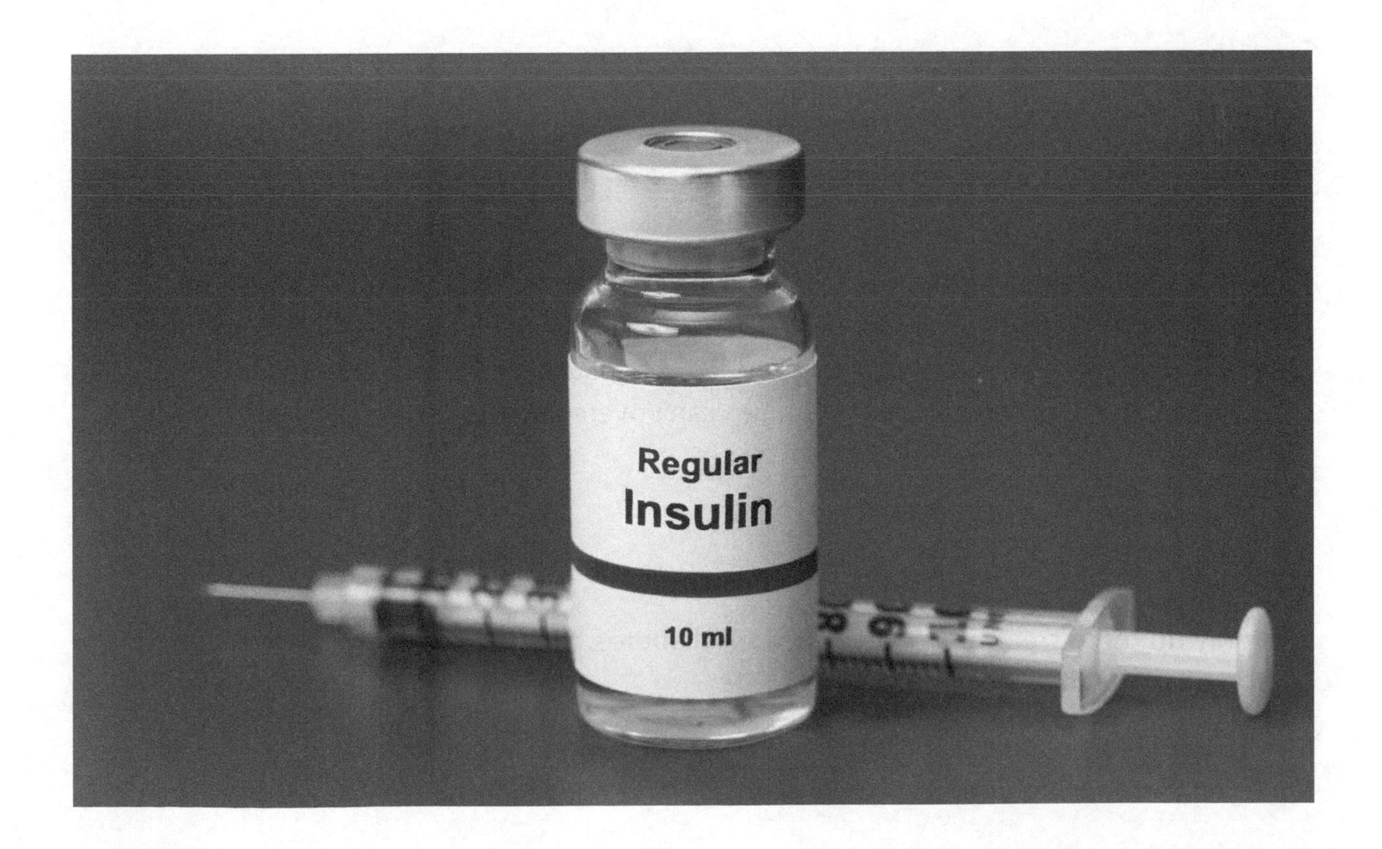

The body regulates insulin levels perfectly in response to what you eat. Any attempt to replace this autonomic control causes major problems in the long run. The use of synthetic insulin disrupts the body's natural homeostasis. It forces your body to shut down its own production of insulin which ultimately causes you to become a true Type 1 diabetic.

Again, synthetic insulin does nothing for the root cause of diabetes and only makes things worse.

Just look at the list of side effects below of what insulin therapy can do to your body:

- Nausea
- Headache
- Heart palpitations
- Blurred vision
- Numbness around the mouth
- Tingling sensation in the fingers
- Muscle weakness
- Irritability
- Loss of consciousness
- Skin reactions (redness, itching, swelling, or rash)
- Body swelling
- Weight gain
- Hormonal imbalance
- Pancreas stops making insulin naturally
- Amputation
- Cancer
- Even death!

NOTE

If you do decide to continue using insulin injections, please read the bonus book about the benefits of using natural insulin. Natural insulin is much safer, and the only reason it isn't commonly prescribed is because it can't be patented. In other words, the pharmaceutical companies can't overcharge for it.

Not only do these treatments not cure your diabetes, the "solutions" aren't even effective at prolonging your life.

The *Veterans Affairs Diabetes Trial* (6) followed two groups of veterans with Type 2 diabetes. One group controlled blood sugar with drugs, and the other didn't. The results? The group with controlled blood sugar had the same risk of heart attacks and dangerous complications as the group not controlling blood sugar.

Diabetes medications won't improve or extend your life.

Medicine isn't supposed to cause more problems than it solves. But that's exactly what modern medicine does. If you're still not convinced, keep reading.

Fabricated Results

Every day Americans are subjected to a barrage of advertising by the pharmaceutical industry. They feature beautiful people enjoying themselves in the great outdoors, pitching the benefits of so-called breakthrough treatments.

But are any of these benefits true? Aren't the pharmaceutical drugs tested? Aren't there studies proving they're safe and effective?

The pharmaceutical industry sponsors 90% of published clinical trials.

Just tell me who's funding the study, and I'll tell you the result … before they even start.

It's clear there is a deep conflict of interest in Big Pharma sponsoring trials on their own drugs. Industry-sponsored trials are four times more likely to produce positive results than independently run experiments.

Producing positive results is clearly not left to chance. Some trials are manipulated by comparing a new drug to inadequate doses of another useless drug. Trial patients are selected by the ones most likely to react well to the given experimental medication.

Many of the trials that fail to show positive results or too many dangerous side effects are simply buried.

For example, take the anti-depressant drug Reboxetine. All the evidence suggested Reboxetine was safe and effective. Later it was found that out of seven trials conducted, only one had positive results. (7) Guess which one they published?

This is just one example; all drug companies operate like this. You just can't trust the results drug companies give. Their decisions are based on profits.

Most so-called studies aren't based on real scientific truth anymore.

The truth is that most pharmaceutical drugs don't work. In fact in most cases, you would probably do better without taking anything at all.

Do Current Diabetes Treatments Work?

No. The current treatments just don't work. You may think that the medication they're giving you will help your condition, but the reality is very different. And you already know this happens if you've been diabetic for some time.

Typical Progression of Diabetes Using Medical Treatments

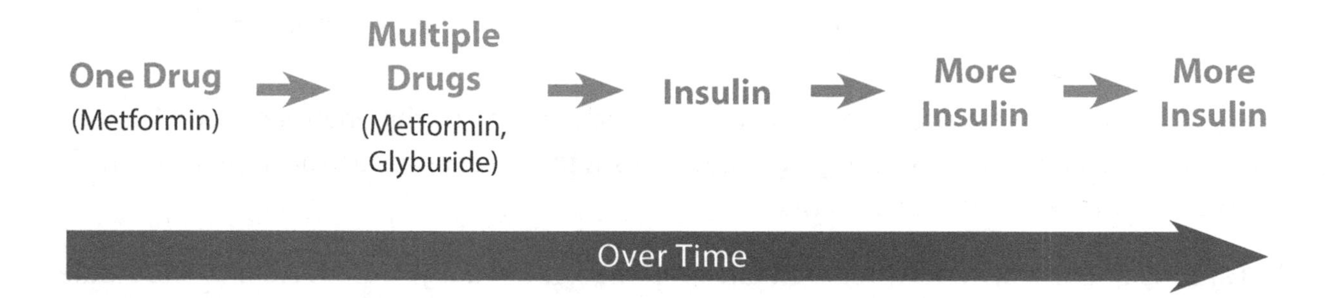

When you're first diagnosed, your doctor puts you on a single medication. And in the beginning, this actually improves your blood sugar levels. But over time, no matter what drug you take, the effects eventually wear off.

So you end up on a second medication or a third medication as your doctors does his best to stabilize your sugar. This pretty much happens to everybody.

Eventually, you end up on a little bit of insulin ... then more insulin ... then more and more insulin.

The people on the fewest drugs are the ones doing better. And the ones on a lot of insulin are the ones with severe diabetes.

So the fact is, over the years and despite what everyone tells you, your diabetes is just getting worse and worse and worse.

So whether your sugar goes up or down from the medication they prescribe, your diabetes is actually getting worse. And multiple studies have proven this.

The UKPDS (United Kingdom Prospective Diabetes Study) (8) was a huge study undertaken in the UK to see if intensive blood glucose lowering in Type 2 diabetes would prevent organ damage over the long run.

Although the drugs were certainly successful at lowering blood sugar levels, they were unable to find any evidence that taking drugs reduces heart attacks or strokes, decreases the likelihood of leg amputations, or improves life expectancy.

Not only did they find that current diabetic treatments don't work, they also discovered that they caused an increased risk of hypoglycemia and weight gain.

Still don't believe drug companies have been lying about the benefits and results of their drugs? Let's just look the lawsuits.

Lawsuits

Here is a list of the 20 biggest lawsuits against the drug companies. (9) There are literally thousands of lawsuits and settlements that I couldn't list in this book. The amount of corruption in the industry is appalling.

YEAR	COMPANY	SETTLEMENT	VIOLATIONS
2012	GlaxoSmithKline	$3 Billion	• Failure to disclose safety data • Paying kickbacks to physicians
2009	Pfizer	$2.3 Billion	• Doctor Kickbacks
2013	Johnson & Johnson	$2.2 Billion	• Doctor Kickbacks
2012	Abbott Laboratories	$1.5 Billion	• Illegal Promotion
2009	Eli Lilly	$1.4 Billion	• Illegal Promotion
2001	TAP Pharmaceutical	$875 Million	• Medicare Fraud • Doctor Kickbacks
2012	Amgen	$762 Million	• Illegal Promotion • Doctor Kickbacks
2010	GlaxoSmithKline	$750 Million	• Poor Manufacturing Practices
2005	Serono	$704 Million	• Illegal Promotion • Doctor Kickbacks
2008	Merek	$650 Million	• Medicare Fraud • Doctor Kickbacks
2007	Purdue Pharma	$601 Million	• Illegal Promotion
2010	Allergan	$600 Million	• Illegal Promotion

YEAR	COMPANY	SETTLEMENT	VIOLATIONS
2010	AstraZeneca	$520 Million	• Illegal Promotion
2007	Bristol-Myers Squibb	$515 Million	• Medicare Fraud • Doctor Kickbacks • Illegal Promotion
2002	Schering-Plough	$500 Million	• Poor Manufacturing Practices
2006	Schering-Plough	$435 Million	• Medicare Fraud • Doctor Kickbacks • Illegal Promotion
2004	Pfizer	$430 Million	• Medicare Fraud • Doctor Kickbacks • Illegal Promotion
2008	Cephalon	$425 Million	• Illegal Promotion
2010	Novartis	$423 Million	• Doctor Kickbacks • Illegal Promotion
2003	AstraZeneca	$355 Million	• Medicare Fraud
2004	Schering-Plough	$345 Million	• Medicare Fraud • Doctor Kickbacks

Government Protection?

What about the government, you ask? Doesn't the Food and Drug Administration (FDA) step in and make sure diabetes drugs and treatments are safe and effective?

Well … that's what it was first created for, but today, it doesn't work anything like that anymore. Pharmaceutical companies have been spending millions of dollars lining the pockets of corrupt politicians in order to keep the drugs flowing.

In fact, most of the top executives at the FDA either worked for Big Pharma in the past or were offered high paying jobs right after their term.

Listen. It's easier to believe what you've been told and follow everyone else rather than think for yourself. This is part of human nature. We want to believe that what the drug companies and government tells us about diabetes is true. Unfortunately, most of it is isn't.

This disinformation is driven into people's minds to such an extent that hearing anything different sounds crazy to them.

If people knew the truth, these industries would lose huge profits because the financial "health" of these operations depends on them having complete control about what the public knows about their own nutrition and health.

Unfortunately, you just can't trust the nutritional information provided by the government anymore. We have to start listening to our bodies.

Diabetes is all about the money, and the pharmaceutical companies are making a killing off of your suffering. Drugs and insulin therapy used to be your only option, but neither is a good option.

In the next chapter, I'll show you a new science. One that is not driven by profits, but instead, one that is driven to put an end to all of the pain and suffering caused by diabetes.

PART 2

THE DIABETES CURE

CHAPTER 3

THE BREAKTHROUGH DISCOVERY

In the next few chapters, you'll learn how a series of breakthroughs led to the discovery of the true cause of diabetes – something the medical industry has suppressed for years.

It all started when a colleague of mine sent me an email of a study he came across. At the time, I was struggling for answers. I had made some progress on my own, but I was stuck. And then I read this.

Obesity Surgeon Finds the Cure

The study was written by a professor from Newcastle University. Dr. Roy Taylor runs their Diabetes Research Group, and his research will change the lives of millions of diabetics.

Although he's met a lot of opposition, he's found a way to publish a paper in a respected medical journal. The first few times he tried to publish this study, he was turned down. Most people didn't believe the results.

Even he didn't believe it at first. As a medical student, you're told that people with Type 2 diabetes get steadily worse and eventually need insulin. Everyone sees diabetes as a progressive and incurable disease.

What makes the resistance to Dr. Taylor's research so surprising is that for years it's been known that Type 2 diabetes can be reversed through extreme calorie restriction – most notably through gastric bypass (weight loss) surgery.

Dr. Taylor first learned about the link between gastric bypass surgery and diabetes in the 1980s when he visited a surgeon named Walter Pories. Gastric bypass surgery is where they use a clamp to reduce the size of your stomach so you get full easier and don't eat as much.

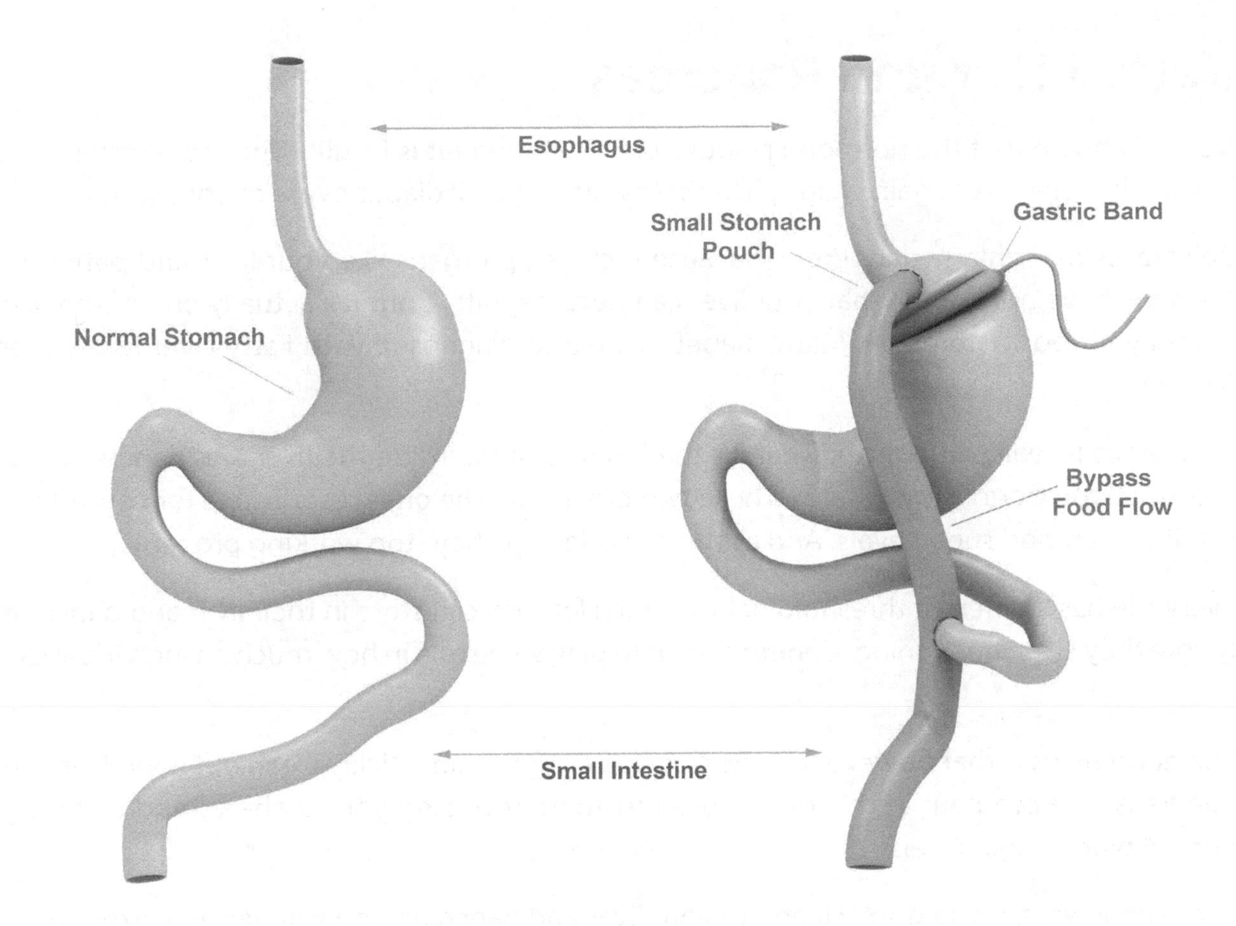

Dr. Pories had been studying weight loss surgery on obese patients. One of those studies followed 608 extremely obese patients for 14 years.

The results of gastric bypass surgery on weight loss were spectacular and more than just weight loss. Patients also saw significant improvements in their health including lower blood pressure, improvement in sleep, and a huge drop in their risk of dying from heart disease.

But to Dr. Taylor, there was one thing of particular interest – of the 608 patients in the study, 311 had pre-diabetes or full Type 2 diabetes. And what he discovered shocked him.

For most of these patients, their blood sugar levels returned to normal shortly after surgery!

Their diabetes cleared in just days, and most of the patients left the study as non-diabetics. They no longer had to take their diabetes medication, even those on insulin.

Even more impressive is that 14 years later in a follow up study, 83% of the former diabetics still had normal blood sugar levels. They were cured!

The only problem was that weight loss surgery is not an easy option. There are serious complications when things go wrong, from diarrhea to infections and even death. In addition, it didn't work in all cases. About 20% of the patients still had diabetes despite having bypass surgery. Still, Dr. Taylor knew he was on to something.

Fatty Liver and Pancreas

It's well known that the hormone responsible for storing fat is insulin. The more insulin you have, the easier it is to gain weight. That's why most Type 2 diabetics are overweight.

Belly fat is particularly dangerous because it clogs up organs like your liver and pancreas. You may have not known that your liver can become "fatty", but it's actually one of the first places your body stores fat. Many diabetics are also diagnosed with Fatty Liver Disease or NAFLD.

Dr. Taylor's research suggested that it's the buildup of fat inside the liver and pancreas that causes all the trouble in diabetes. These two organs are the ones responsible for controlling insulin and blood sugar levels. And as the fat builds up, they stop working properly.

Everyone has a different threshold of how much fat they can store in their liver and pancreas before they stop functioning. Genetics seem to play some role in how much an individual can store.

The good news is that however clogged up you are, you can quickly clean out your liver and pancreas (the program in this book does just that), reversing your diabetes and restoring normal blood sugar levels.

The bad news is, if you don't clean out your liver and pancreas, you will not only experience the complications of diabetes, you may also permanently damage these organs.

The New Castle Study

As soon as Dr. Taylor realized the significance of this discovery, he came up with a calorie-restricted diet that mimicked what patients ate after gastric bypass surgery. That way, the fat could be cleared out of the liver and pancreas without surgery.

First, he needed to be able to measure exactly what was happening to the levels of fat in the liver and pancreas of his patients. For that, he used an MRI machine that happened to be available at the university.

Next, he needed funding, but with most funding coming from pharmaceutical companies these days, he needed to look elsewhere. They didn't want a cure to jeopardize their profits. Lucky for him, he found a nonprofit organization to give him enough money for a small study of 14 patients.

These patients were taken off of their diabetes medications and given a strict, calorie-restricted diet for eight weeks.

As the fat clogging up their livers melted away, their symptoms improved. And by the end of the eight weeks, many of them saw drastic improvements in their fatty livers. Just look at a MRI scans from one of those patients.

BEFORE **AFTER**

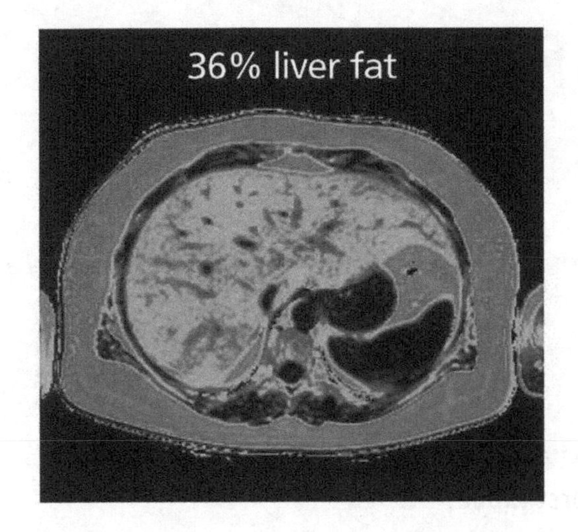

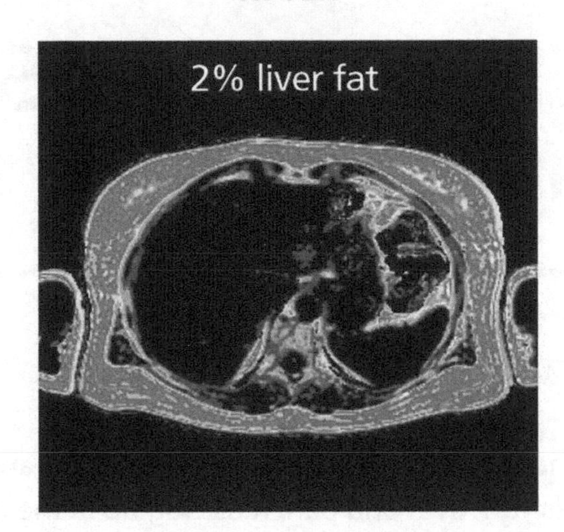

100%

0%

For the volunteers that stuck to the diet for the full eight weeks, they lost an average of 33 pounds and 5 inches off their waistlines. Even more impressive, 100% of these patients saw their blood sugar returned to normal. Now these people were pre-diabetics or folks that were recently diagnosed. So Dr. Taylor created a second study to find out whether this would work with long-term, Type 2 diabetics.

The results were almost as incredible!

The second study was published in 2015 and tested 29 people who had Type 2 diabetes for either 4-8 years or more than 8 years. Again, they found that those who stuck to the diet got great results.

In this study, 87% of the group who had been diabetic 4-8 years and 50% of those who had diabetes for more than 8 years completely reversed their diabetes. Their blood sugar was back to normal without any medication.

Dr. Taylor's discovery has shown that Type 2 diabetes can be reversed in very motivated people. But I knew there was more to this story. Not all of the patients reversed their diabetes, and I couldn't expect people to starve themselves to get these incredible results.

CHAPTER 4

THE TRUE CAUSE OF DIABETES

In the last chapter, we learned that fat in the liver and pancreas was connected to diabetes. But why does your liver and pancreas clog up in the first place?

This stumped me for years. I had my mind wrapped up around sugar being the main culprit. All of my research focused around sugar, but sugar alone wasn't the answer. I kept researching until I discovered the information I'm going to share with you today.

I can't stress how important this is. This discovery is a true medical breakthrough that can end Type 2 diabetes for good.

People just need to forget the medical establishment's narrative that Type 2 diabetes isn't reversible. (They just want to peddle more drugs.)

Once you understand the true root cause, you'll see how easy it is to fix.

Diabetes isn't the lack of insulin in your body or insulin resistance as you've been told. That's only part of the story. The true cause of diabetes is something completely different.

Before we get to that, I want to explain something very important.

The human body is one of the most complicated and incredible things in the entire universe. It's so complex that we may never fully understand how it all works. Nothing you can take or do is going to cure your diabetes. The only way to cure diabetes is to give the body what it needs so it can cure itself.

To understand the true root cause, we are going to have to get a little more detailed on how your cells use energy. I've done my best to simplify my ideas, but if you don't understand a concept, don't worry. The solution to all of this is super simple, and we'll get to that in Part 3 of this book.

The TRUE Cause of Diabetes

This is by far the most important factor in developing diabetes, so read carefully.

Your body is made up of trillions of cells, and each one of them needs energy to survive – just like you do. Your cells feed primarily off sugar in the form of glucose.

Everything you eat ultimately gets converted into glucose and sent into your bloodstream.

In a perfectly healthy environment, glucose is easily absorbed through the cell wall. The cells don't require insulin to absorb glucose (this is a myth). (10) (11)
Now here's the **true cause** of diabetes "they" don't want you to know.

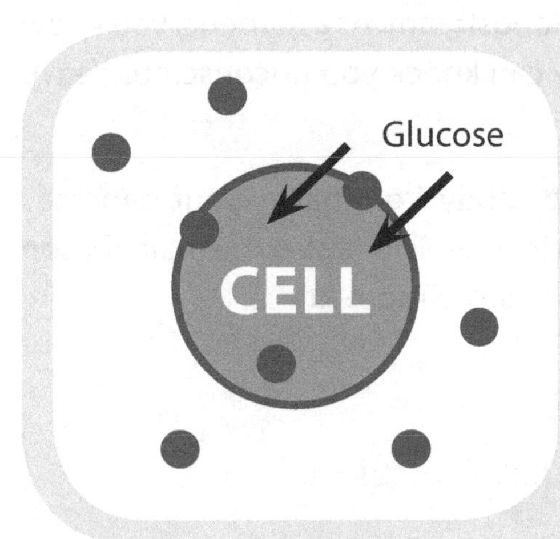

Healthy Glucose Metabolism

Healthy cells can easily absorb glucose from the bloodstream.

Insulin is not required for this to take place as the medical Industry has tricked you into believing.

When you eat a typical meal, say pork chops and potatoes, you take in a good amount of fat and glucose – fat from pork chops that might be fried and glucose from the broken-down carbohydrates from the potatoes.

Now, if you took some of you blood after this meal and put it into a centrifuge (a machine that spins things really fast), you'd separate the red blood cells from everything else. And what you'll see floating at the top is a murky layer of fat. The fat you ate for dinner is now traveling through your arteries.

If your body has a high amount of fat floating in your blood (lipids), your cells get coated with a layer of fat. This makes it impossible for glucose to enter the cell. Cells become weak, and sugar builds up in your blood stream because it's not being absorbed by the cells.

(Insulin resistance can be created in laboratory animals by injecting fat directly into their liver blood supply)

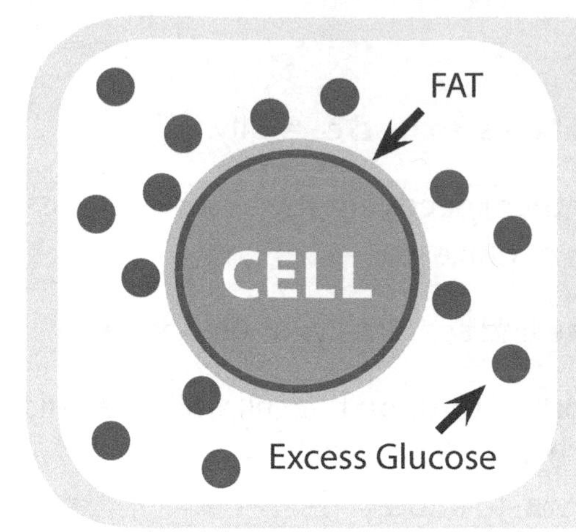

High Lipid Glucose Metabolism

High blood lipids (FAT) are very sticky and coat the outside of your cells, making it very difficult for the glucose to be absorbed by the cells.

This is why your blood sugar spikes, and you still feel tired. High blood sugar is dangerous, and that's where insulin comes in.

Insulin is how your body deals with excess glucose in the bloodstream. As a diabetic, you know that high blood sugar levels can be very dangerous. They can knock you unconscious, leave you in a coma, or even cause death!

In order to deal with this excess glucose and protect your body from harm, your pancreas creates insulin which then grabs excess glucose and stores it as fat. This is also the main reason diabetics tend to be overweight. Insulin forces your body to store more fat.

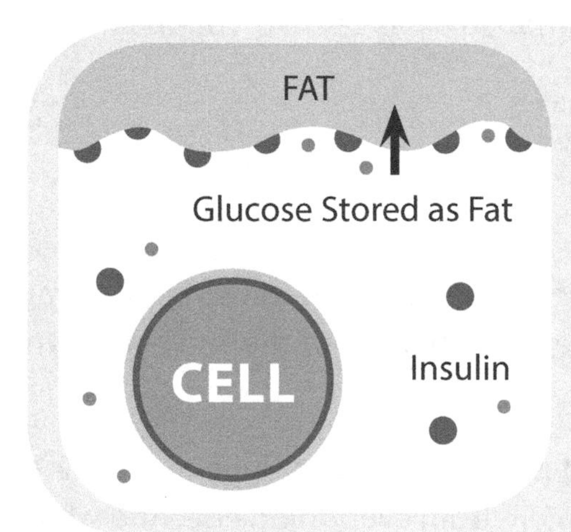

Insulin Function

The body releases insulin to get rid of excess glucose in the bloodstream. Without insulin, your body would go into shock.

While taking insulin injections does help the body recover from the damage caused by high blood sugar, it doesn't address the underlining cause.

Since the way you've been eating has caused your cells to be chronically covered in fat and your blood filled with sugar, your pancreas has to produce an excessive amount of insulin day after day.

TO CLARIFY – THE TRUE CAUSE OF DIABETES IS TOO MUCH FAT AND TOO MUCH SUGAR IN YOUR BLOODSTREAM AT THE SAME TIME.

It's not that either fat or sugar is bad for you. It's when you eat excessive amounts of both with every meal.

For example, you could eat a diet that's pure sugar, and as long as you eat little to no fat, your diabetes would reverse. In fact, a raw, fruit-only diet does exactly that, and it's super high in sugar. It even works with Type 1 diabetics.

The same goes for a diet high in fat. You can eat all the bacon and butter you want as long as you don't eat any sugars or carbohydrates at the same time.

We'll get to exactly what to eat to reverse your diabetes in the next section, but for now, let's connect what we just learned to what we discovered in the last chapter.

An Overworked Liver

Your liver receives 30% of the blood circulating in your system every minute. It's your very own chemical plant, helping remove harmful toxins and distributing and storing essential nutrients for your body.

Your liver's role in diabetes is the one most ignored by doctors. I bet you didn't know that your liver plays a bigger role in leveling your blood sugar than your pancreas plays.

In fact, when doctors at John Hopkins University autopsied diabetes patients, they found that only 2% had degenerated pancreases, while 98% had degenerated livers!

The liver serves two important functions for diabetics. First, your liver can remove a tremendous amount of excess glucose from your bloodstream.

But maybe even more important is its ability to remove excess fat! Yes, the same fat that coats your cells and prevents them from using glucose.

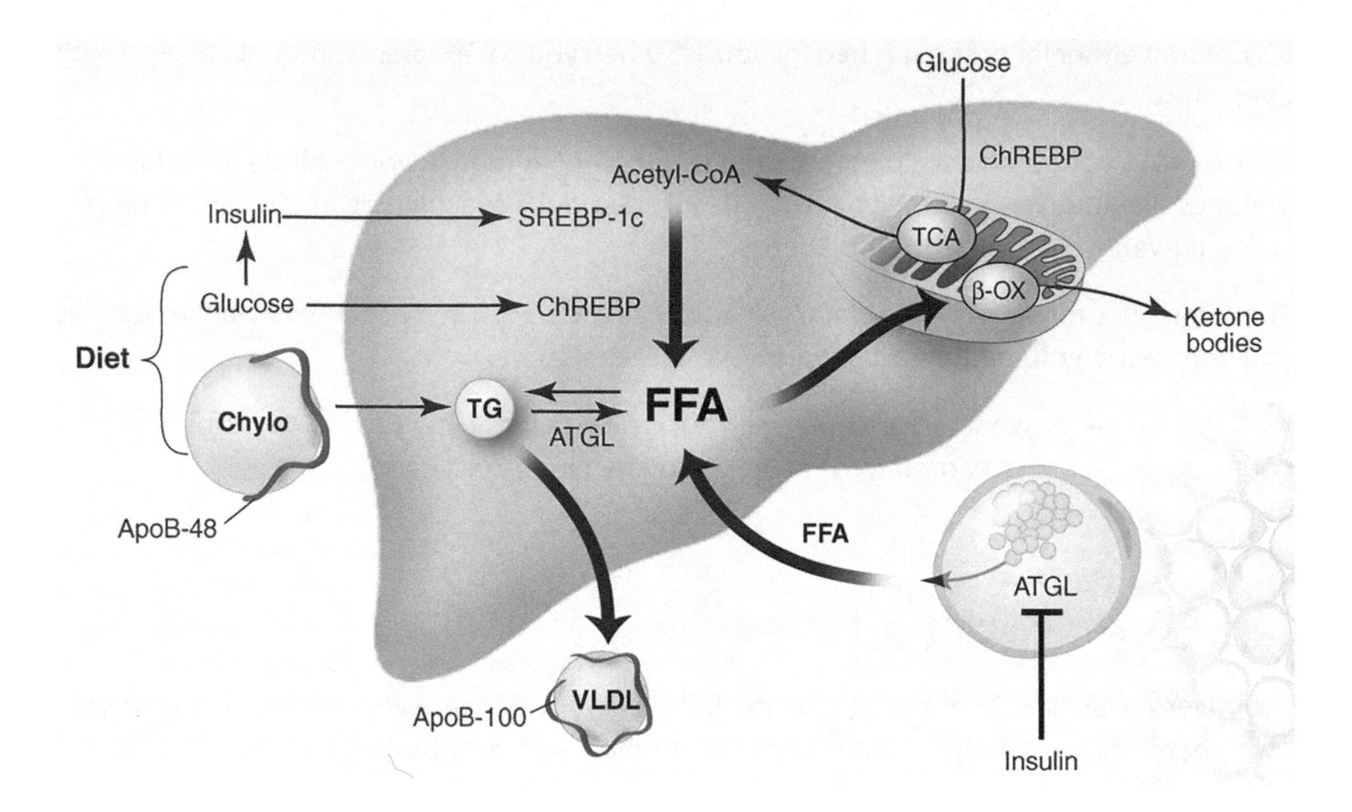

As I stated before, the true cause of Type 2 diabetes has to do with high levels of fat lipids in the blood with high levels of glucose. If your liver isn't functioning properly, it won't be able to do its job of removing fat and sugar from the blood.

Unfortunately, your liver was never designed to deal with our modern diet. And I'm here to tell you, the way you are eating is the cause of your diabetes. But don't worry; you don't have to give up the foods you love. As you'll soon learn, you just need to make a few simple adjustments.

Why Your Liver and Pancreas Get Clogged

As I've said before, the true cause of diabetes is too much fat AND too much sugar at the same time. Eating the Standard American Diet year after year covers your blood cells in fat, and your excess blood glucose gets out of hand.

Your body only has one choice – release more insulin. As you learned earlier in the book, Type 2 diabetics have too much insulin.

Insulin's primary role is to signal the liver to store excess sugar as fat. And since the easiest place for your body to store fat is your liver, that's exactly why it gets clogged up so quickly. As soon after that, the pancreas gets clogged as well.

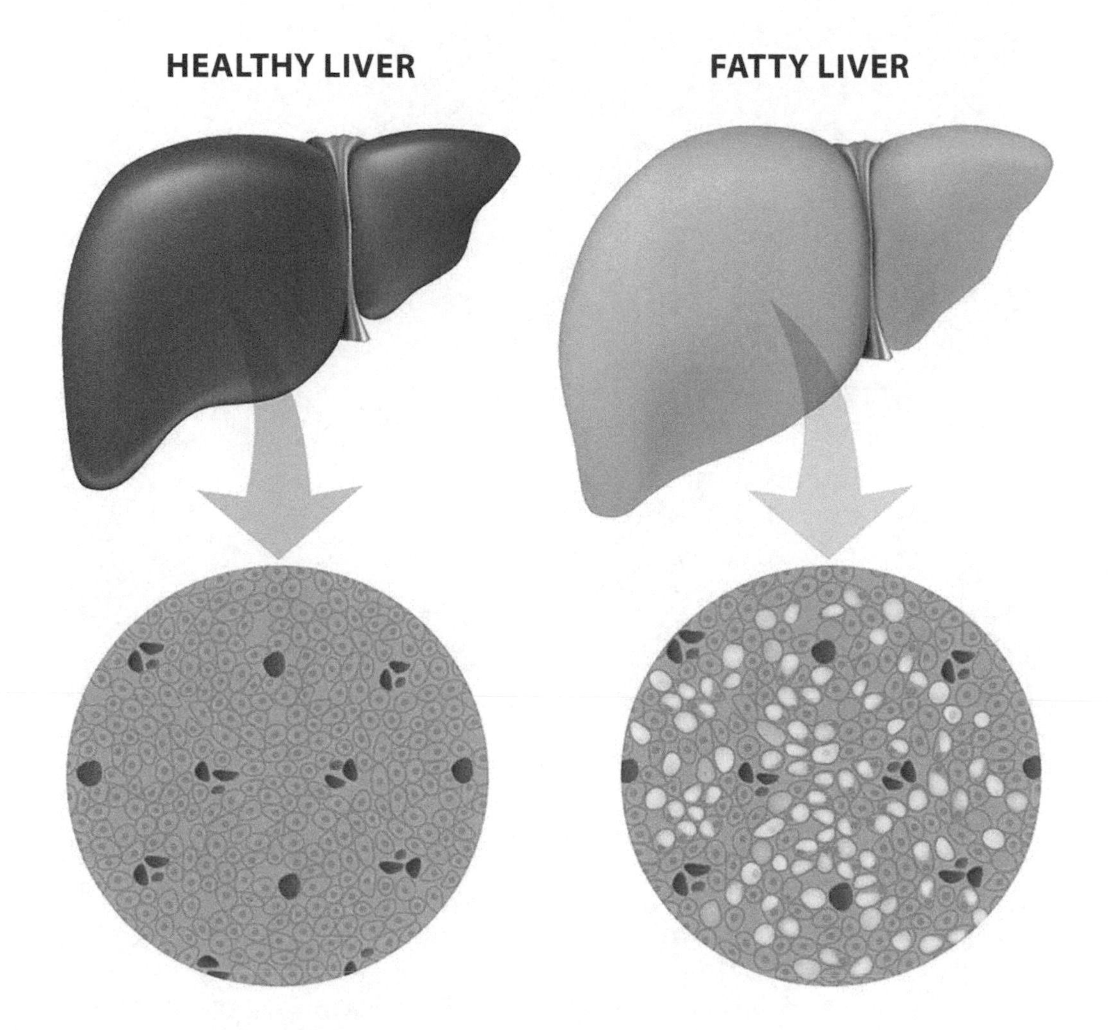

As you can see in the illustration above, a fatty liver looks very different from a healthy liver. And they function very differently as well.

So the key to reversing diabetes is cleaning out your liver and pancreas and getting them working normally again. Start by eating the right way, so they never get clogged up again.

Giving Type 2 diabetics more insulin is insane. Excess insulin is the reason your liver clogs up in the first place. This is why diabetics get worse and worse once they start taking insulin.

You don't have to go down that path anymore. You don't need to suffer through the horrible complications of diabetes, because you know the true cause ...

A fatty, non-functioning liver and pancreas are caused by too much sugar and fat in the bloodstream at the same time.

But how do you fix all this? Easy, by following Diabetes Free! In the next part of this book, we'll go into The Diabetes Free Program, and I'll give you a 3-step plan anyone can follow to completely reverse diabetes. So let's begin.

PART 3

THE DIABETES FREE PROGRAM

REVERSING DIABETES IN AS LITTLE AS 11 DAYS

So far, I've explained the background to the current diabetes epidemic, the standard medical treatments and their dangers, and the new science that completely reverses diabetes for good!

Now it's time to get to the specifics of the Diabetes Free Program. I've spent my entire adult life studying human health, and I promise you, this program works!

Actual Results

"I am writing to report the good news. I followed the Diabetes Free Program with the liver cleansing and pancreas healing. I cannot believe the result is so good and true. In less than 4 weeks, my blood sugar dropped from 154 to 75. I deeply appreciate David Pearson's effort in helping diabetes sufferers."

DIABETES FREE SUCCESS STORY – FELICE

Just follow this easy, 3-Step Program, and you'll be shocked at how quickly your blood sugar stabilizes and your symptoms disappear. Follow these simple steps and watch in amazement as you become Diabetes Free!

STEP 1

Cleanse Your Liver & Pancreas

The proper functioning of your liver and pancreas is crucial to reversing diabetes. In this first step, you'll use a powerful combination of herbs in a delicious shake that gently cleanses and reactivates the cells in your liver and pancreas.

STEP 2

The Diabetes Free Diet

The Diabetes Free Diet is simple. We've broken down the diet into easy-to-understand guidelines, so you can't go wrong. You'll get a choice of two diets – the "FastTrack" version and one for those who prefer to go "Slow & Steady".

STEP 3

OPTIONAL - Get Some Exercise

For diabetics who want to accelerate their results, adding some light exercised such as walking is a great idea. Exercise helps burn up excess sugar and clear out deposits of fat from the liver and pancreas.

Once you start seeing results, remember to send us a testimonial so we can share it with others and showcase the benefits of this powerful program.

What are you waiting for? Let's get you started!

IMPORTANT!

DO NOT STOP TAKING YOUR MEDICATION OR INSULIN.

CHECK YOUR BLOOD SUGAR OFTEN AND WORK WITH YOUR DOCTOR TO ADJUST THE DOSAGE OF YOUR MEDICATION OVER TIME.

Before You Start

I've been critical of doctors in the earlier sections of this book, but I'm not anti-doctor. Most are good, hard-working people who have just been misinformed through what they've learned in medical school. (Hint: Big Pharma's sponsored curriculum)

So it's important to talk to your doctor before starting this program. This is especially true if you are on any medication. You'll need their help to safely taper off these drugs.

As a general rule, if your blood sugar drops to normal or below normal for a few days, you will need to lower the dose of your medication. Ask your doctor for guidelines in advance with specific blood sugar targets as well as how much to drop the medication.

I wish I could give you my recommendations on how to cut your medication without seeing you in person, but that just isn't possible. So you'll have to work with your doctor.

While many doctors will be delighted that you are taking responsibility for your health, some may be unimpressed. If yours is in the second group, it may be time to find another doctor.

While some may attempt to do this program without the help of a doctor, I strongly advise against it.

Use extra caution if any of the following applies to you:

» You are on insulin or a medication other than metformin (if you are, you'll need to reduce those medications quickly to avoid your blood sugar from dropping too quickly).

» You are on blood pressure or blood-thinning medication (you'll most likely have to reduce or come off them completely).

» You have moderate or severe retinopathy (if so, you should have extra screening for six months following the completion of this program).

» You are pregnant or breast-feeding (may be best to wait until after).

» You have a significant psychiatric disorder or a form of epilepsy (talk to your doctor).

» **NOTE:** You should not do this program if you ar-e recovering from major surgery.

Having said that, there are a few things to keep in mind before you get started.

TREATING HYPOGLYCEMIA IF YOU ARE UNCONSCIOUS

Diabetics are always at risk of losing consciousness if blood sugar falls very low. If you measure your blood sugar often, and work with your doctor to lower your medication, this should not be a problem.

However, to be on the safe said, it's a good idea to have a Glucagon Emergency Kit handy that someone can use if you become unconscious from very low blood sugar.

Glucagon is sold in pharmacies. It's a syringe filled with a sugar like substance. More information visit: *www.lillyglucagon.com*

Tests You Should Have Done

Before undergoing any new treatment, it's always a good idea to visit your doctor to get a clean bill of health. I recommend basic blood work to look for anything serious.

Make sure to ask for the following tests:

» A1C (long-term blood sugar levels)

» CBC (complete blood count)

» Kidney function tests (urea and electrolytes)

» Liver function tests (including GGT)

» Blood lipids profile

It's also a good idea to measure your weight and waist size. Remember to take before-and-after pictures so you can fully appreciate how much of a change you've gone through in eight short weeks.

Measuring Your Fasting Glucose

If you're like most diabetics, you probably check your blood sugar before each meal. If you don't, it's time to start.

I know how painful pricking your finger can be, but with Diabetes Free, you will find your blood sugar dropping quickly, and you'll need to adjust accordingly. This is especially true if you're taking insulin.

BLOOD GLUCOSE LEVELS	
Normal Range:	70–100 mg/dl (3.9–5.5 mmol/l)
Pre-diabetes:	101–125 mg/dl (5.6–7.0 mmol/l)
Diabetic:	Over 125 mg/dl (over 7.0 mmol/l)

Use the Tracking Guide that came with your Diabetes Free Package. Make sure you record your glucose levels right before each and every meal. You'll use the results as motivation and to show your doctor that it's time to reduce or eliminate your prescription meds.

How to Check Your Blood Sugar Levels

1. Wash and dry your hands; using warm water may help the blood flow.

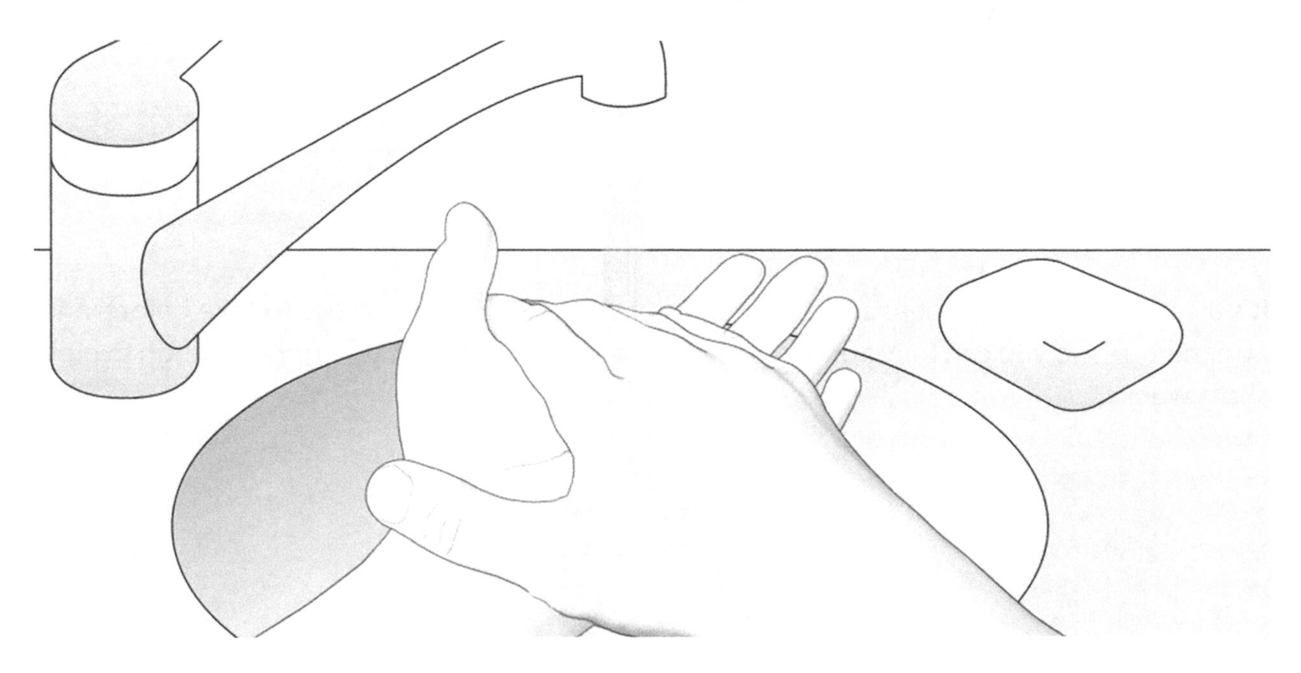

2. Turn on the meter and prepare a test strip as outlined in your owner's booklet.

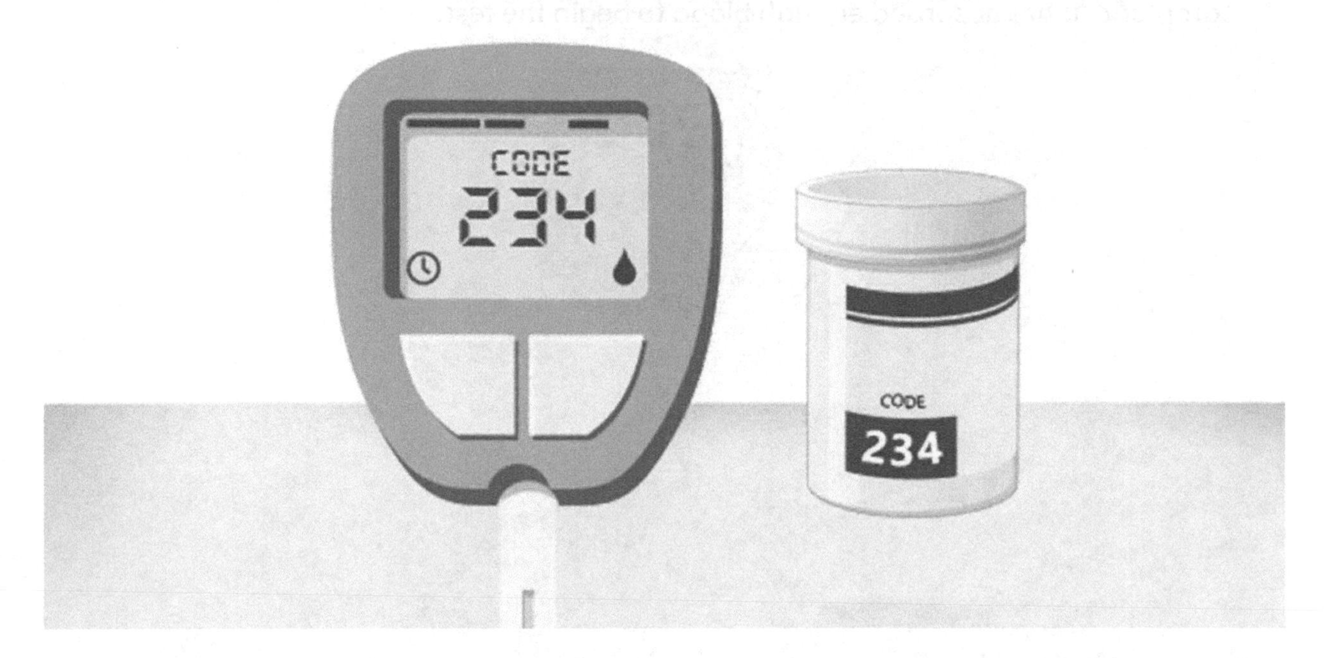

3. Choose your spot; don't check from the same finger all the time. Follow the manufacturer's instructions to prepare the lancing device and get a drop of blood from the side of your fingertip or other approved sites.

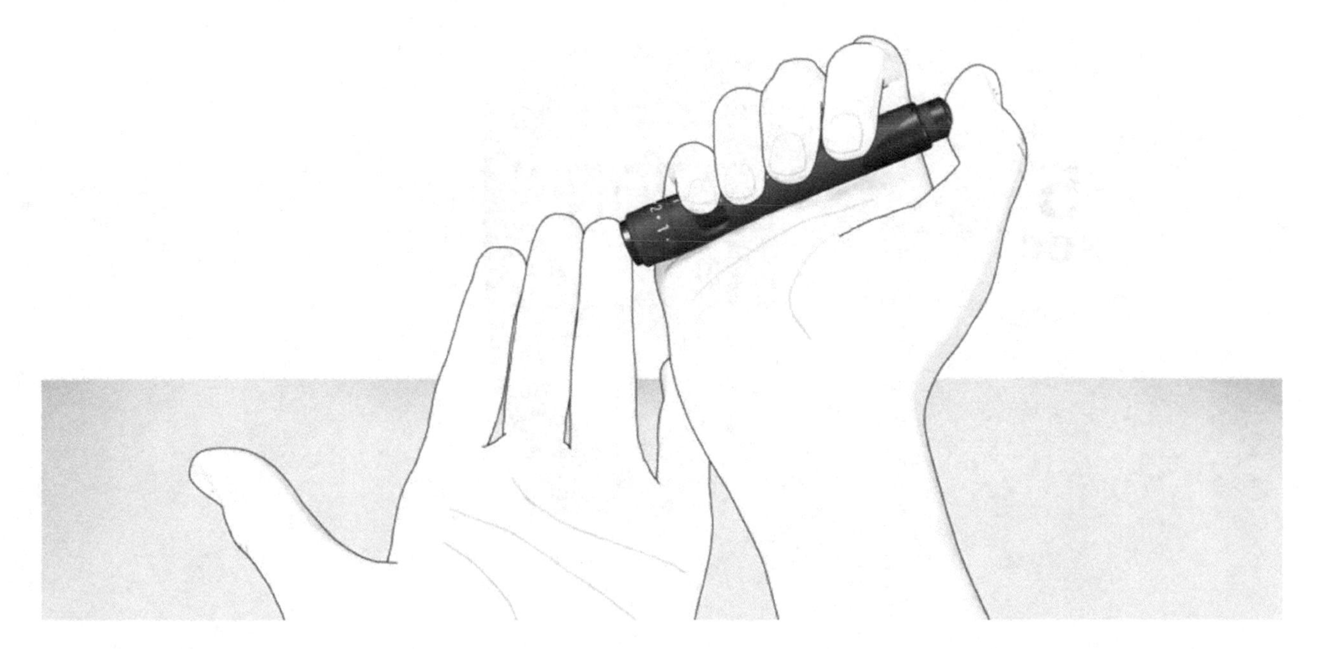

4. Check your blood sugar by touching and holding the test strip opening to the blood drop until it has absorbed enough blood to begin the test.

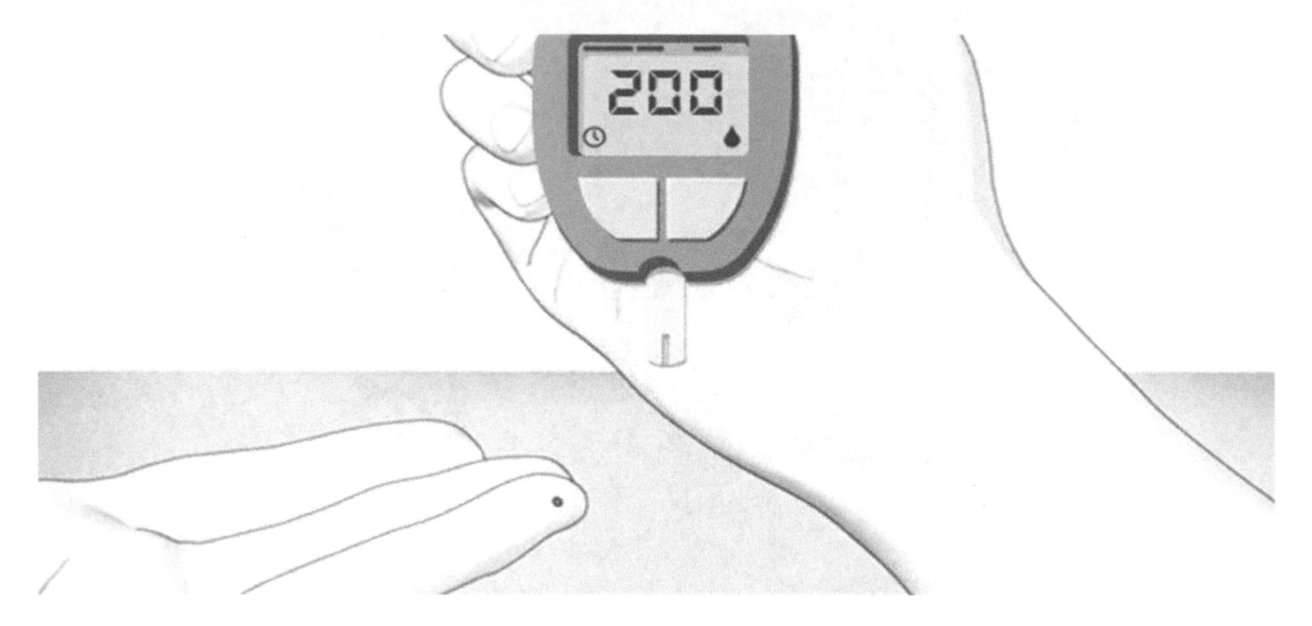

5. View your test result and take the proper steps if your blood sugar is too high or low based on your healthcare professionals' recommendations.

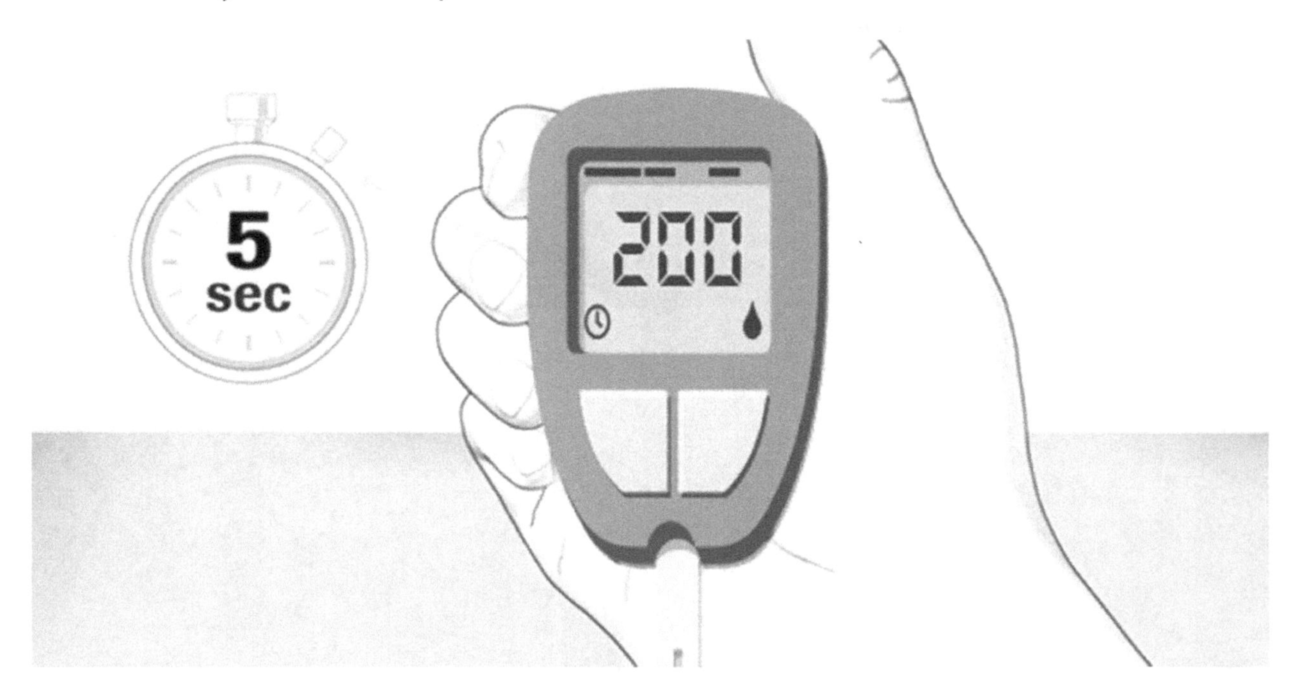

6. Discard the used lancet properly.

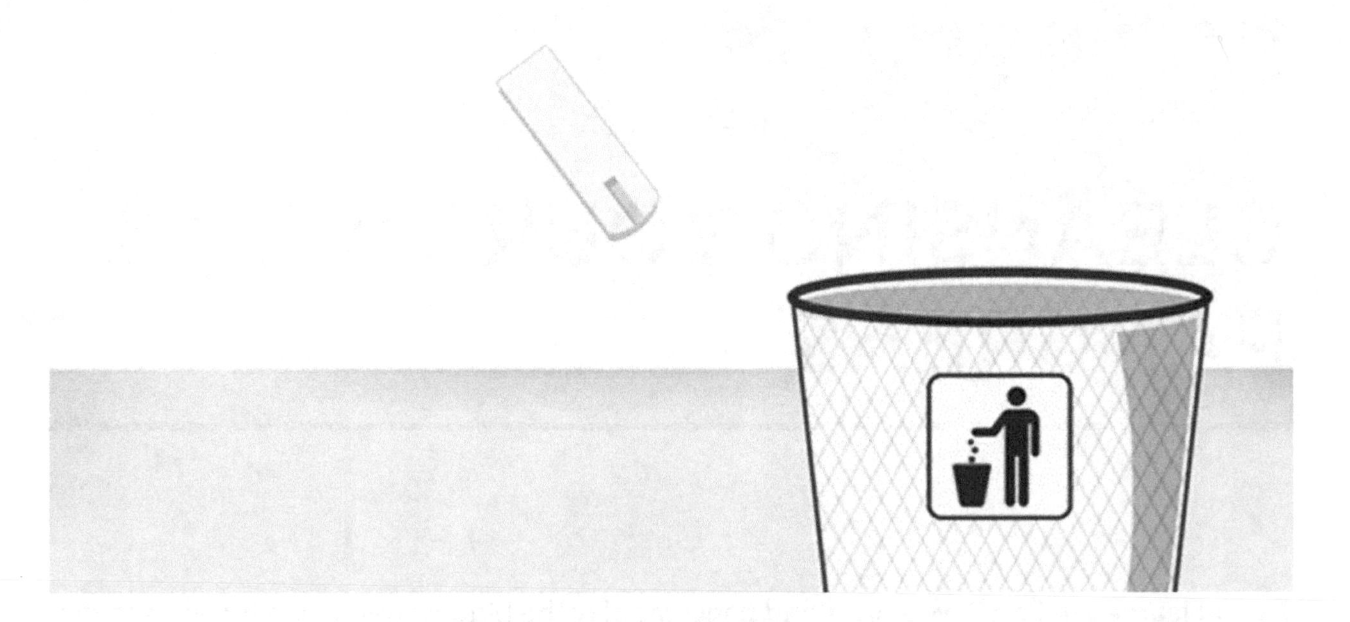

7. Record the results in the Diabetes Free Tracking Guide, so you can review and analyze them later.

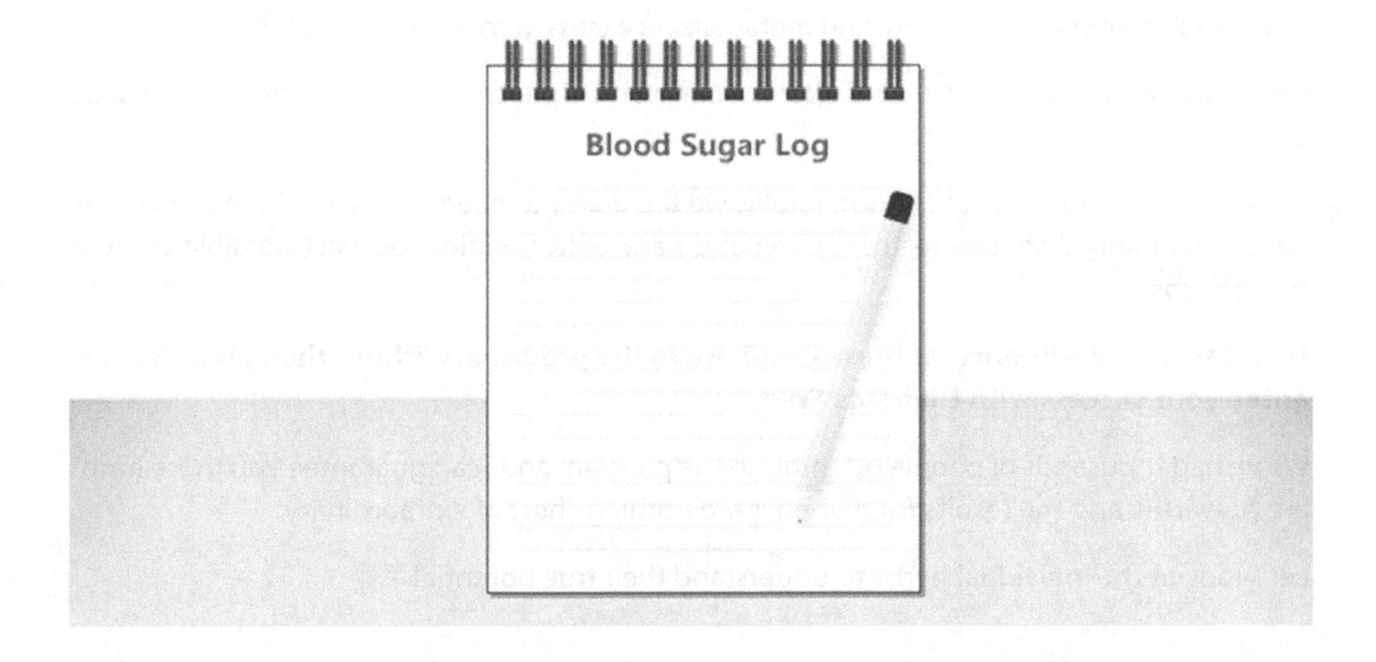

CHAPTER 5

CLEANSING YOUR LIVER & PANCREAS

As you learned in Part 2, your liver and pancreas play the biggest role when it comes to diabetes. You also learned that the way to reverse diabetes is to cleanse your liver and pancreas and restore their normal function.

The reason we cleanse your liver and pancreas is so they can start working properly, cleaning out the fat in your blood stream, and metabolizing excess glucose, 24 hours a day.

Unfortunately, if you already have diabetes, your liver and pancreas have been clogged for quite some time.

In order to restore their function naturally, we are going to need the help of some powerful herbs. For many diabetics, restoring liver and pancreatic function just isn't possible without these herbs.

I can't stress how important these herbs are to the program. Without them, I can't guarantee your success with Diabetes Free.

We've had thousands of people go through the program and I can guarantee you these herbs are powerful, and the results for diabetics are nothing short of extraordinary.

Let's look at the individual herbs to understand their true potential.

INGREDIENT	PROPERTIES
Jie Geng Extract (Platycodi Radix)	Jie Geng improves glucose homeostasis by enhancing insulin sensitivity. The active saponins can lower cholesterol levels in the liver and promote bile acid secretion.
Licorice Root Extract (Glycyrrhizae Radix)	Licorice root contains substances with an anti-diabetes effect. These amorfrutins not only reduce blood sugar, they are also anti-inflammatory and very well tolerated. Licorice root is effective at reducing ALT and AST concentrations in the liver.
Schizandrae Chinese Fruit Extract (Schizandrae Fructus)	Schizandra is used in China to regulate blood sugar levels, reduce high cholesterol, and improve overall health. It also improves liver function and provides relief from Fatty Liver Disease.
Shepherd's Purse Extract (Capsella Bursa)	Shepherd's Purse stimulates circulation, helps stabilize blood sugar levels, and eliminates liver congestion.
Astragalus Membranaceus Bunge Extract	This extract improves blood sugar levels and protects the liver from cellular dysfunction and liver fibrosis.
Lycium Fruit Extract (Lycium Barbarum)	Lycium fruit has been used for centuries in China for its anti-aging properties and longevity enhancements. It's also used in the treatment of diabetes as it protects and tones the liver.
Chicory Extract (Cichorium Intybus)	Chicory has a long history of herbal uses and tonic effects on the liver and digestive tract. It is used widely as a hypoglycemic.
Polygonati Rhizoma Extract	Rhizome extract reduces fasting blood glucose, decreases glycosylated hemoglobin (GHb), and improves glucose tolerance.
Fenugreek Seed Extract	Fenugreek seeds are high in soluble fiber. The seeds have a number of health benefits, one of which is lowering blood sugar by slowing down digestion and absorption of carbohydrates.
Balloon Flower Root Extract (Platycodon Grandiflorus)	Balloon Flower Root is used as an anti-bacterial and an anti-fungal, and it has shown anti-tumor activity in animals. It lowers blood sugar and helps flush out liver parasites.
Solomon's Seal Extract (Polygonatum Biflorum)	Solomon's Seal contains chemicals that decrease blood sugar levels and harmonize the liver while helping to remove fat deposits.

INGREDIENT	PROPERTIES
Mulberry Leaf Extract (Morus Alba)	Mulberry leaf has been traditionally used to treat diabetes by numerous cultures around the world. Evidence from human studies shows that it significantly reduces the rise in blood sugar that occurs after a meal and helps the liver at the same time.
Dioscorea Japonica Thunberg Extract	Dioscorea Japonica improves muscular strength and increases stamina. It also strengthens liver function and increases immune system resistance. It is a medicinal plant that is known to have anti-diabetes actions.
Neem Leaf Extract	Neem enhances insulin receptor sensitivity and seems to work well for Type II diabetics. It balances the liver and reverses Fatty Liver Disease.

All of these ingredients come together to form the Diabetes Free Shake.

How & Why The Diabetes Free Shake Works

The Diabetes Free Shake is based on over three decades of research and combines these discoveries into a powerful, yet delicious shake. It works synergistically at three levels to provide liver and pancreatic cleansing, healing the underlying problem that caused the disease in the first place. Simple put, this is how it works:

1. First, several ingredients work together to manage glucose levels that spike from each meal you eat. This quickly stabilizes your blood sugar levels to prevent any further damage to your liver or pancreas. This is what makes the Diabetes Free Shake work so quickly.

2. Next, key ingredients reactivate liver function and balance the Insulin producting receptors in the pancreas. This allows your own body to manage your blood sugar effectively.

3. Finally, and most importantly, the remaining ingredients work together to clear out existing fat deposits blocking your liver and pancreas from working effectively. This takes some time, depending on how clogged they are, which is why we recommend taking the Diabetes Free Shake for at least 3 months.

How To Make The Diabetes Free Shake

I've tried to make this as simple as possible, but you need all these herbs to make the formula work. You can find these ingredients for purchase on the Internet, or even at your local health food store.

Make sure all ingredients are either organic or wildcrafted. It's important all these herbs are of the highest quality or they may not effective:

» Jie Geng Extract 60mg (Approx. 1/32 tsp)
» Licorice Root Extract 60mg (Approx. 1/32 tsp)
» Schizandrae Chinese Fruit Extract 60mg (Approx. 1/32 tsp)
» Shepherd's Purse Extract 200mg 60mg (Approx. 1/32 tsp)
» Astragalus Membranaceus Bunge Extract 60mg (Approx. 1/32 tsp)
» Lycium Fruit Extract 60mg (Approx. 1/32 tsp)
» Chicory Extract 60mg (Approx. 1/32 tsp)
» Polygonati Rhizoma Extract 60mg (Approx. 1/32 tsp)
» Fenugreek Seed Extract 60mg (Approx. 1/32 tsp)
» Balloon Flower Root Extract 60mg (Approx. 1/32 tsp)
» Solomon's Seal Extract 60mg (Approx. 1/32 tsp)
» Mulberry Leaf Extract 60mg (Approx. 1/32 tsp)
» Dioscorea Japonica Thunberg Extract 60mg (Approx. 1/32 tsp)
» Neem Leaf Extract 60mg (Approx. 1/32 tsp)
» Stevia Powder 1000mg (Approx. 1/2 tsp)
» Cocoa Powder 4000mg (Approx. 2 tsp)

Directions:

Add all ingredients into a 8oz glass of water. Mix thoroughly with a spoon. Drink immediately. Take the shake 3x per day, right before each meal.

Ideally, you should continue to take the shake everyday even after your blood sugar stabilizes using the duration chart above. In doing so, you will continue cleaning and balancing your body so you never have to deal with diabetes again.

Supplier Disclaimer

Before making the shake please research all herb brands and suppliers. Unfortunately, we cannot guarantee the effectiveness of the Diabetes Free Program when using ingredients sourced from unknown suppliers for the following reasons:

1. You cannot be certain of the safety of the ingredients (many suppliers use herbs contaminated by pecticides and other toxic chemicals)
2. You cannot be certain about the quality or potency of these products because they may or may not have been tested for strength and effectiveness.
3. You cannot be certain the herbs have not been damaged due to high speed manufacturing practices. (High heat destroys these ingredients)

How Much Do You Need?

This is a tough question since I don't know your medical history, how long you've had diabetes, or how closely you'll stick to the recommended diets. Having said that, I've put together some guidelines based on what I've learned while working with former diabetics who have gone through the program.

CURRENT HEALTH	RECOMMENDED SUPPLEMENT DURATION
Pre-diabetic Or Diabetic For Less Than 3 Years	3 Months
Diabetic For 3-7 Years Or Currently On insulin	3-6 Months
Diabetic For More Than 7 years And On insulin	6-12 Months

If you have any reservations about herb suppliers or making the Shake yourself, then we recommend you use Sugar Balance. This is a supplement we produce that contains all of the ingredients listed above at the highest quality and potency.

Why We Created Sugar Balance

When we first started sharing The Diabetes Free Program, we used to recommend specific third-party herb suppliers to help support the amazing results of the program. Unfortunately, over time, we began to recieve customer feedback on the effectiveness of the program.

Upon research, we discovered the quality of these herbs from the suppliers was very inconsistent (due to lower quality ingredients to increase profits) and these led to customers not seeing the results they expected.

This did not sit well with us.

Our corporate mission is to bring health and wellness alternatives to the masses – a revolutionary Diabetes Free System with products that ACTUALLY work, are of the highest quality and at a price point that consumers can afford. Naturally, we couldn't continue to recommend a substandard product to our customers.

Without any good alternatives, we decided to take matters into our own hands. We spent countless months sourcing the highest quality ingredients available and made sure our supplements were manufactured to the highest standards possible.

Research

All of these ingredients have been clinically tested and proven effective in double blind studies. They are the result of decades of research from leading universities and reserach firms around the world.

This is the real deal. It's been thoroghly tested for safety and effectiveness in thousands upon thousands of patients.

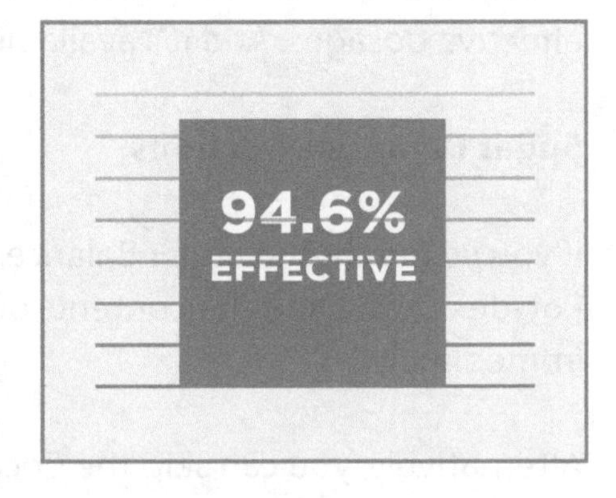

This stuff works. In fact, when combined and used in a study, 94.6% of diabetics saw drastic improvements within 3 months of use.

If you're the type of person who likes to dig into research, you can view the papers and studies that lead to the discovery of the Diabetes Free Program listed in the reference section at the end of this book.

After almost a year of our own internal research and testing, we created Sugar Balance.

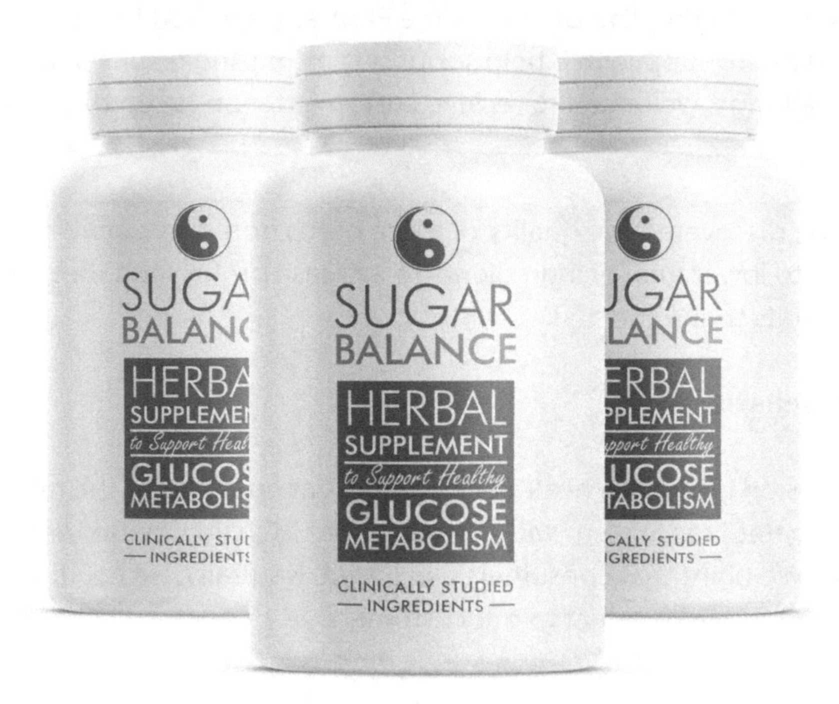

Not only does Sugar Balance contain all the ingredients needed at effective dosages, it's also the most cost effective formula.

Sugar Balance is a product that we proudly and confidently stand behind. It contains the highest quality ingredients and has the strongest potency, so our customers can get the results we promise.

Sugar Balance is the only guaranteed way to get all the specific herbs used for the shake at effective dosages. And it's available exclusively for Diabetes Free customers.

Sugar Balance Directions:

If you've purchased Sugar Balance, making the shake is even easier. Just mix the Cocoa Powder, Stevia and the contents of 1 pill into 8oz of water. Mix thoroughly and drink immediately.

Alternatively, you can skip the Cocoa and Stevia and just take the pill before each meal. Most customers find it much more convinent to swallow a pill then to hassle with mixing the shake. Both methods are just as effective.

How To Get It

If you did not order a bottle of Sugar Balance with your purchase of The Diabetes Free Program, you can still get it.

FOR A LIMITED TIME: New customers are eligable for a 30% discount if you order within 7 days of purchasing The Diabetes Free Program.

Note: It's made in small batches to ensure potency and quality, so sometimes they run out of stock. It's best to order as soon as possible, so you aren't delayed starting the Diabetes Free Program. You can place your order on the site below:

www.GetSugarBalance.com/Discount

CHAPTER 6

THE DIABETES FREE DIET

Now that you have some powerful herbs cleansing and reactivating your liver and pancreas, it's time to add a special diet that accelerates healing even further.

Using the herbs and diet together is the one-two punch that is the magic behind the Diabetes Free Program. With these two steps, your diabetes will be reversed in no time.

The Diabetes Free Program diet is divided into two phases.

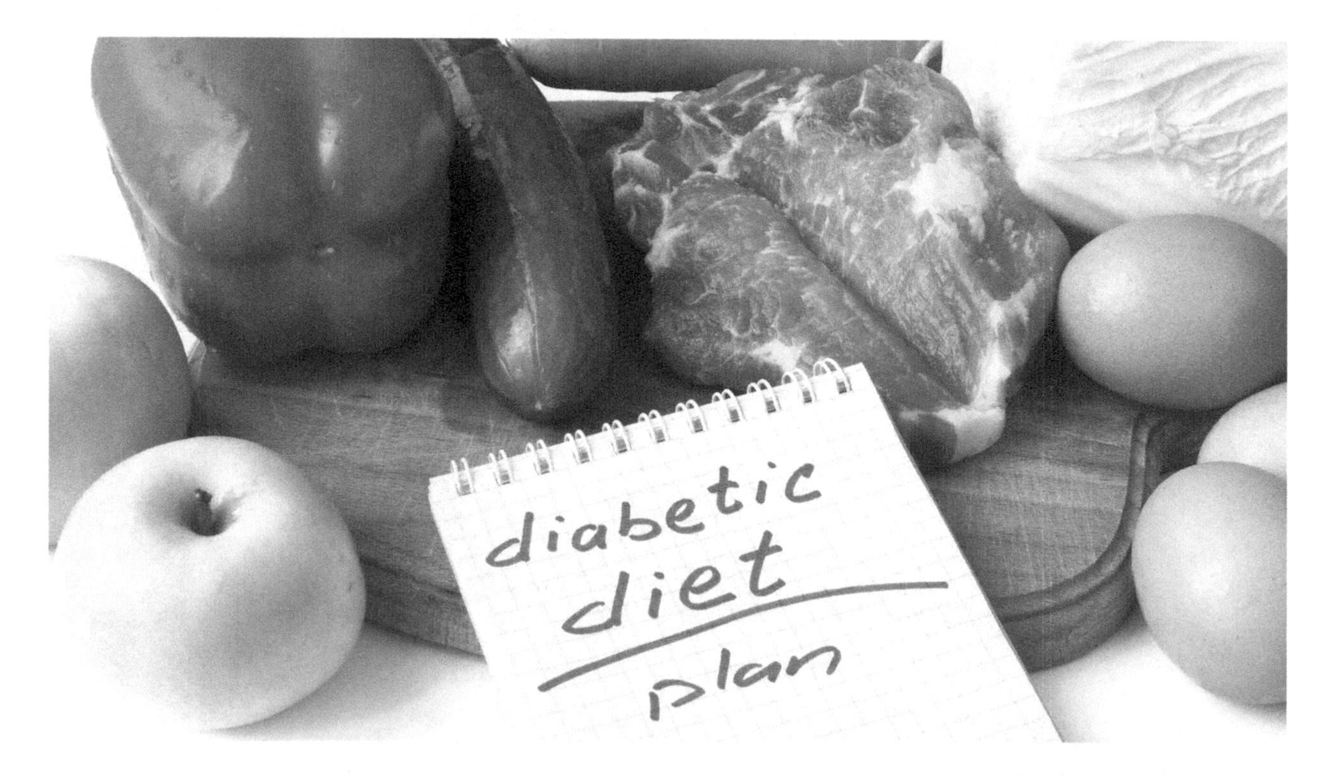

The first phase is a short, intense cleanse that enables your body to unclog your liver and pancreas. It's critical that you complete this phase to get the full benefits of this program. I'll give you a few options to make this as easy as possible.

The second phase starts after your blood sugar drops to non-diabetic levels. This is more of a guide to which foods to eat for the rest of your life. Even though you'll no longer be diabetic, you don't want to eat the foods that caused you to get diabetes in the first place.

Otherwise, a few years down the road, you may become diabetic again. If you're thinking you'll be on a restricted diet your whole life, don't worry. You'll still be able to enjoy all the foods you love, plus this new way of eating will help you lose unwanted weight, boost your energy levels, and have you feeling better than ever before!

Let's get started.

How Have Our Diets Changed?

Many, many years ago, our great ancestors led a very different life. Although our digestive systems haven't evolved much since then, it is important to note that our diets have changed tremendously. In this section, we will explore how this affects your body, and more specifically, how it damages your liver and pancreas.

What Did Early Humans Eat?

Although our diet evolved over millions of years, I want to focus on three major shifts that got us where we are today.

It's now known that early humans ate a diet almost identical to our closest genetic relatives – the great apes. In fact, studies have shown that 99.4% of our DNA is identical to animals such as the bonobo chimpanzee. They ate a diet that was primarily fruit. This makes sense because early humans lived in tropical regions to stay warm since they didn't wear clothes yet, and fruit is plentiful and delicious in such areas.

What's important to note is that their diet was almost entirely carbohydrate-based because of the sugar in fruit. This means they ate a lot of sugar and little to no fat. Yet none of these early humans were Type 2 diabetics.

Our first shift happened nearly 40,000 years ago. At this point and as populations grew, some humans began to migrate north into colder areas. Fruit became rare so in these locations that they were forced to expand their diet to include animal products for survival. They ate every part of the animal (especially the fat) and used their fur to make clothes.

The significance here is that they ate a lot of fat but very little sugar. Again, none of them were diabetic.

The second shift happened about 10,000 years ago. This is when humans started to eat grains. Grains are full of carbohydrates which eventually turn into simple sugars. These grains were stone ground and less processed, so they didn't spike insulin as much as the breads we eat today. So even though they ate sugar and fat, their livers were strong enough to keep them healthy.

The third shift happened in the early 1950s. This is when our consumption of industrialized processed foods began, and food quality dropped rapidly. Processed carbohydrates and high fructose syrup have very high glycemic indexes which forces your body to make large amounts of insulin. Just look at how much more sugar we consume each year.

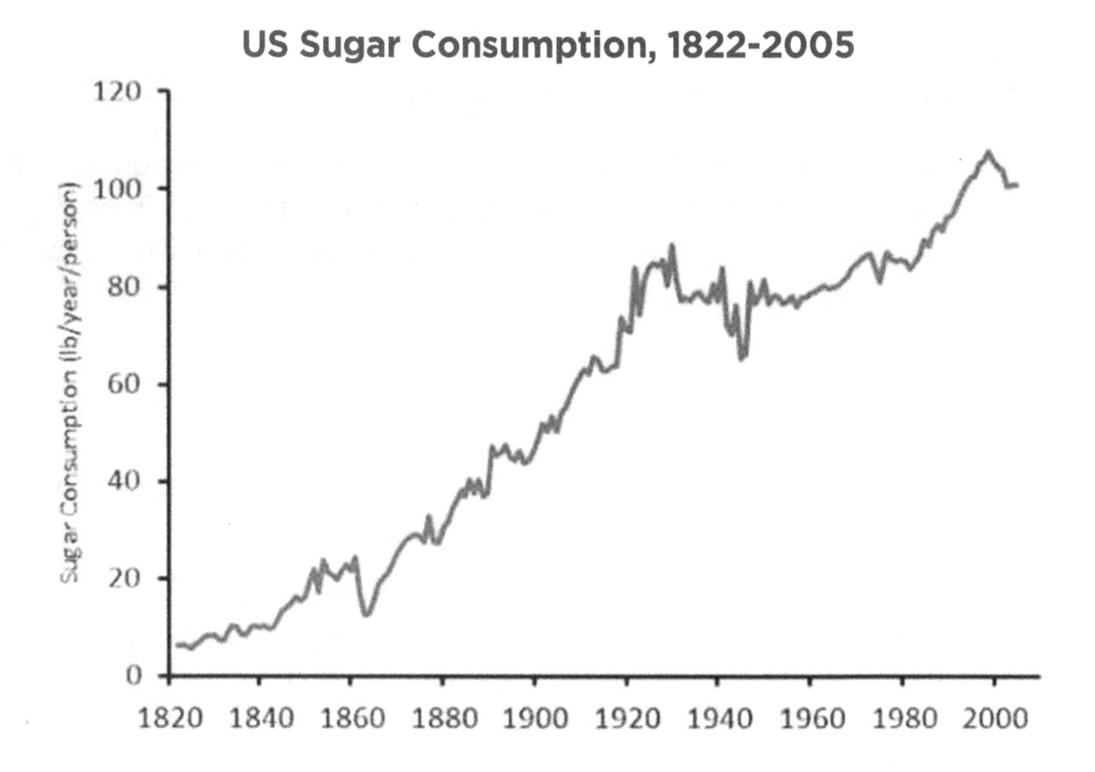

We've gone from five pounds of sugar a year to an astonishing 100 pounds of sugar a year in blink of an eye in human history. This wouldn't have been much of a problem if we didn't also increase our consumption of fat, but that's exactly what happened.

Just look at these statistics:

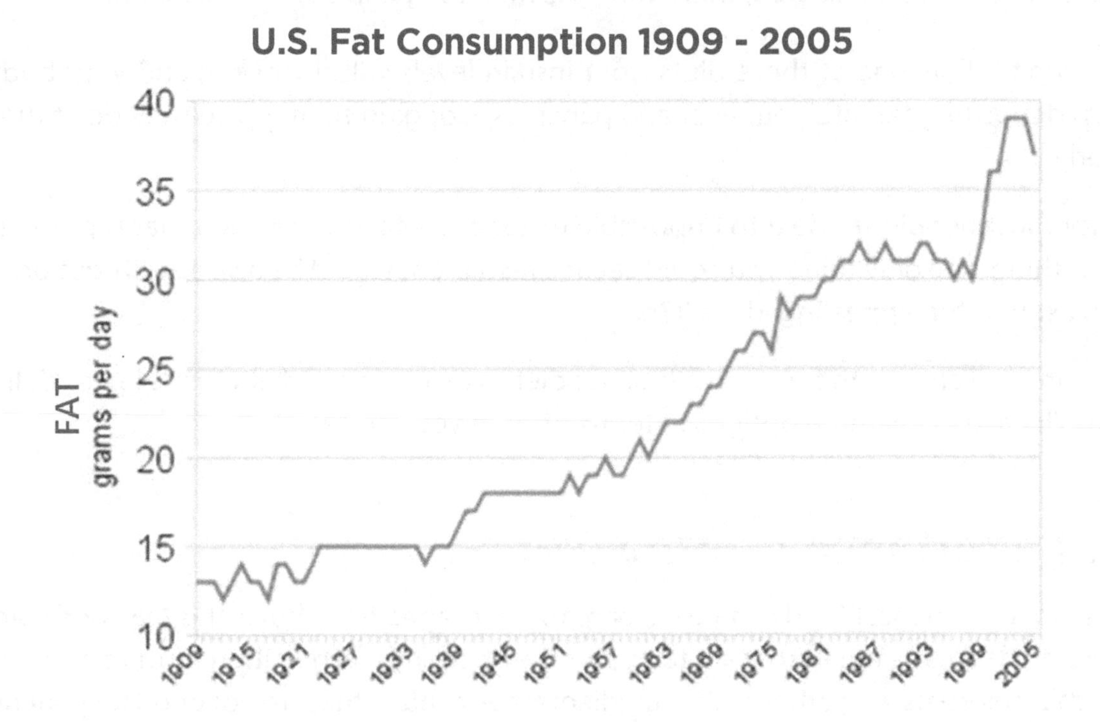

What's important to remember is that our consumption of both fat and sugar has gone up drastically in the last 100 years. Throughout history, there has been a time when we ate so much sugar and so much fat at the same time. Diet is the main reason for the Type 2 diabetes epidemic. No drug will ever change that.

Important Takeaways

Fat/Sugar Balance

As we just learned, for most of human history, we didn't eat fat and sugar at the same time. Our body really wasn't designed to handle how much fat and sugar we now consume each day.

If you remember from earlier chapters, eating fat and sugar at the same time is the main problem. When you eat both at the same time, the cells get covered in fat, and the body needs to release large amounts of insulin to deal with the high blood sugar levels.

Knowing this, if we are to design the perfect anti-diabetes diet, we really only have two options:

1. **Eat a High-Carbohydrate Diet** – Consume large amounts of foods such as bread, pasta, potatoes, fruit, and sugar, and avoid all forms of fat.
2. **Eat a High-Fat Diet** – Consume mostly meat and non-starchy vegetables. This way, even if the cells are coated, there won't be much sugar in the bloodstream.

If you don't follow one of these diets, your insulin levels will skyrocket, and your body will end up depositing fat into your liver and pancreas, clogging them up so they don't function properly.

Now for most people, it's next to impossible to eat a low-fat diet seeing as fat is pretty much in everything. The only thing you could eat at a restaurant would be a salad without dressing. Doesn't sound too appealing, does it?

This is why I've chosen to focus on a high fat diet to reverse your diabetes. It tastes delicious, and you'll have many more options in terms of what you can eat.

The Importance of Whole Foods

It's easy to head to a fast food restaurant or grab a packaged treat, but is this real food? Modern processing has made meals that are tasty, but they lack any real nutrition – not to mention the chemicals, colorants, and other toxic ingredients they contain that are not good for your health.

Instead, it's important to choose whole foods. When you consume a whole food such as an apple instead of apple juice or piece of chicken instead of a nugget, you get it the way nature intended. Eating more whole foods will help anyone get healthier, but that's especially true for diabetics.

First, whole foods contain many more nutrients when compared to processed foods. Many of these vitamins, minerals, and other phytonutrients are required in order for your body to function properly. They're used in every process including creating hormones such as insulin.

Second, whole foods still have all of their fiber. Since it's harder for your body to digest fiber, the amount of glucose released through digestion is slower. This means less insulin and fewer spikes in blood sugar.

Third, whole foods keep you full longer. So instead of getting hungry an hour after you eat, you'll feel satisfied throughout the day. This leads to choosing healthier foods and eating less.

This is why the Diabetes Free diet is built around whole foods.

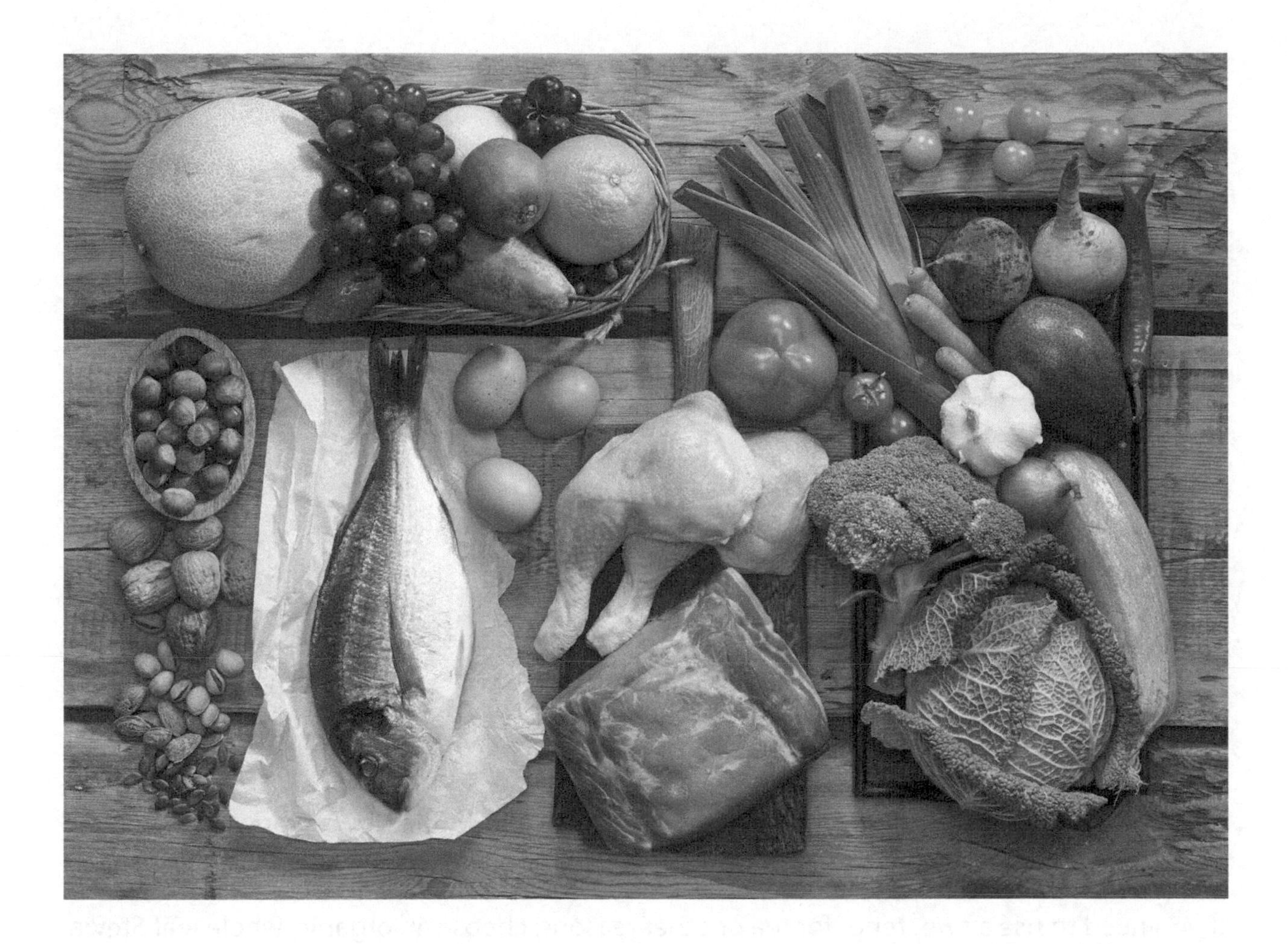

No Diary

There is no diary allowed on this diet at any time. Here's why:

Type 1 diabetes is an autoimmune disease in which the body's immune system attacks and destroys the insulin-producing cells of the pancreas. The American Diabetic Association says that the causes of Type 1 diabetes are not known.

Baloney! There may be different causes, but one cause has been identified: exposure to cow's milk.

Normally this isn't a problem because your body blocks these proteins from entering your bloodstream unless you have a condition called Leaky Gut Syndrome (very common these days).

And research has shown that when proteins found in dairy get into the bloodstream, your body reacts as if it were being attacked by something foreign, so it creates antibodies to protect you.

But what happens is these antibodies don't just attack the dairy proteins. Researchers have identified 17 proteins in dairy that are the same proteins found in the insulin-producing cells of the pancreas.

This means if you happen to have leaky gut (many people do) and consume dairy, you are very likely to become a Type 1 diabetic.

Type 1 diabetes strikes people at any age. It comes on suddenly, can cause dependence on injected insulin for life, and carries the constant threat of devastating complications. And you don't want this.

We know dairy can cause Type 1 diabetes, so it's best to avoid it altogether. That means avoiding all foods that contain diary. Read labels carefully.

No Artificial Sweeteners

There are no artificial sweeteners allowed on this diet. This includes Sweet'n Low, Equal, NutraSweet, Sunett, Sugar Twin, Splenda, The Sweet One and Stevia containing maltodextrin.

Although you may have been told that these are safe for diabetics, the exact opposite is true. No one should ever use these artificial sweeteners. They have been linked to all sorts of serious disease including cardiovascular disease, diabetes and even cancer! Avoid them at all costs, even if you're not diabetic. They are toxic.

Plus, the don't even help your blood sugar levels. In fact, in studies it was shown that people who used artificial sweeteners had more problems controlling blood sugar levels.

If you need to use a sweetener for tea or other reasons, choose an organic, whole leaf Stevia.

Vegetarian Options

Tofu and soy beans are good substitute for those people who want to avoid meat. About half the calories in these products come from vegetable fats, and the balance from varying amounts of protein and slow acting carbohydrates.

They are easy to cook in a skillet or oven. Carbohydrate content should be read from the labels and you should choose the ones with the lowest amounts. Make sure there is no added sugar. Health food stores stock many of these products.

Reverse Diabetes through Fasting

The first phase of the Diabetes Free Program involves fasting. That means periods of time where you're eating very little or nothing at all. New research suggests this is really good for you in general, and it's especially good for your liver.

If we think back to Dr. Taylor's research, we can see very clearly how quickly fasting can clear out the liver. This is a before-and-after picture of a patient's liver through the 8-week fast.

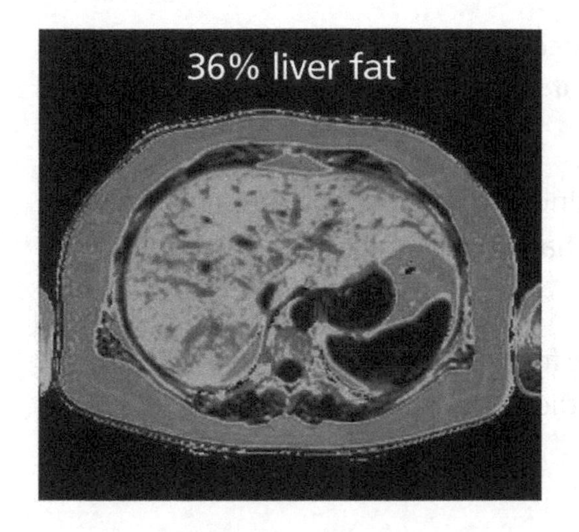

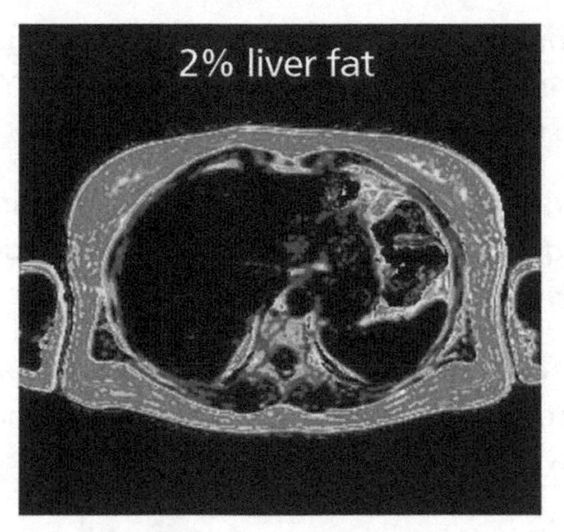

100%

0%

You can clearly see the amount of fat removed during a short but intensive fast. This is critical to the Diabetes Free Program. It's not something you can skip if you want to reverse your diabetes.

When most people hear the word "fast", they worry that it will be very hard to do, and they'll be left starving. But I can tell you from being on many fasts myself, they are very easy to do once you get past the first few days. Your body naturally adjusts and lowers your hunger levels. And as strange as this sounds, you end up having more energy.

If you look to nature, when an animal gets sick, its first instinct is not to eat. Fasting cleanses your whole body, not just your liver. So get started soon, and stick to it!

The Diabetes Free Diet Program

So you've decided to go for it! You've talked to your doctor, cleared your kitchen of tempting foods, and now you're ready to repair your liver and pancreas from the inside out.

If you're pre-diabetic, this diet will stop you from ever developing Type 2 diabetes. If you're already a Type 2 diabetic, this diet is crucial to reversing your condition and returning your blood sugar levels to normal.

To make it as easy as possible, I've given you two options for the fast – a quick but intense 8-week fast and a slower, easier-to-follow 3-6 month fast. You choose what's best for you. Let's go over these diet options now.

Option 1: FastTrack - 800 Calorie/Day (8 Weeks)

The first option is the fastest way to unclog your liver and reverse Type 2 diabetes.

For eight short weeks, you eat 800 calories of food each day and drink plenty of water. That might seem low, but it's not as hard as it sounds. Your body will quickly adjust within days, and you'll no longer feel hungry.

The diet works in conjunction with the Liver Cleansing supplement to completely reverse diabetes as quickly as possible. If you don't already have them, they are available at *www.GetSugarBalance.com/Discount.*

It's very important that you only eat low-carbohydrate foods to get the most impact from this diet. There are many foods that aren't allowed on this diet, so it's easier for me to list the foods that are allowed.

What to Eat & Drink

Here are the simple guidelines for the FastTrack, 800-Calorie Diet:

» For 8 weeks, you will consume a maximum of 800 calories per day.

» The diet will focus on whole foods with an emphasis on non-starchy vegetables, eggs, seafood, and meat.

» You must drink at least two liters of pure water every day (I prefer distilled). If you don't like the flavor, add some fresh squeezed lemon juice.

» You can find delicious recipes near the end of this book. Each recipe is marked with its total calorie count. Eat any combination you want as long as it doesn't add up to more than 800 calories per day. It's okay if it's a little over that.

» You can find more recipes on the web at this site: *www.eatthismuch.com*. Make sure to select paleo and 800 calories as options for the search.

ALLOWED FOODS (YOU CAN EAT ANY OF THE FOODS BELOW AS LONG AS YOU DON'T GO OVER 800 CALORIES PER DAY.)			
All meat	Cauliflower	Celery	Spinach
All poultry	Asparagus	Tomatoes	Brussel Sprouts
All seafood	Mushrooms	Zucchini	Radishes
Eggs	Kale	Onions	Okra
Peppers	Cucumbers	Eggplant	Fennel
Broccoli	Lettuce	Cabbage	Bok Choy
Herbs: Parsley, cilantro, basil, rosemary, thyme, pepper, garlic			
Salt: small amounts of sea salt			
Fats: No added fats other then what is in meat and eggs naturally			

FastTrack Tips

Here are a few tips to make these eight weeks a little easier:

» Try to eat at the dinner table. If you eat on the go or in front of a TV, you're much more likely to eat beyond the point of fullness. While you're at it, avoid watching the food network.

» Eat slowly. It takes time for your body to tell your brain its full. Try putting your fork down after every bite and waiting 30 seconds. And if you get full, stop eating. It's okay to leave some food on your plate.

» Avoid processed foods at all costs. Basically, skip anything that comes in a box, can, or bag. Manufacturers often put chemicals in food to make you hungry.

» Try not to shop on an empty stomach. This will only lead to poor choices.

» If you get hungry, eat some vegetable soup. It's very filling with few calories. It's cheap and practical to make in large quantities.

» Keep tempting foods out of the house and out of sight.

» Weigh yourself often. As you watch the scale drop, you will be motivated to keep going.

» If you must go to a restaurant, eat a healthy meal at home before you go, then get a plain salad and skip the dressing. This way you'll be less tempted to cheat.

» DO NOT drink alcohol on the FastTrack Program. This will delay or even prevent liver cleansing. If you must drink alcohol, choose the Slow & Steady Program instead.

7 Day Sample Meal Plan

DAY ONE

Breakfast: Sunny side asparagus (see page 84)

Lunch: Tuna stuff red pepper (see page 91)

Dinner: Fish & zucchini chips (see page 98)

Snack: Soup of choice (see page 105)

Total Calories: 795

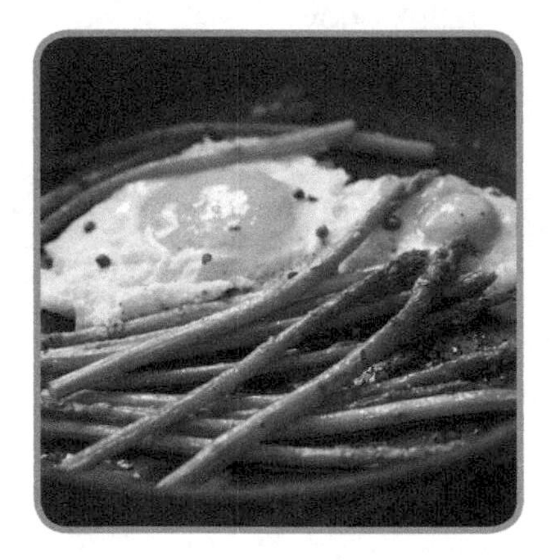

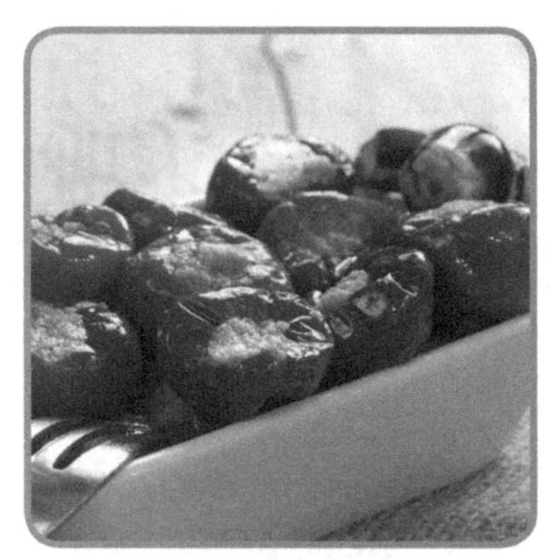

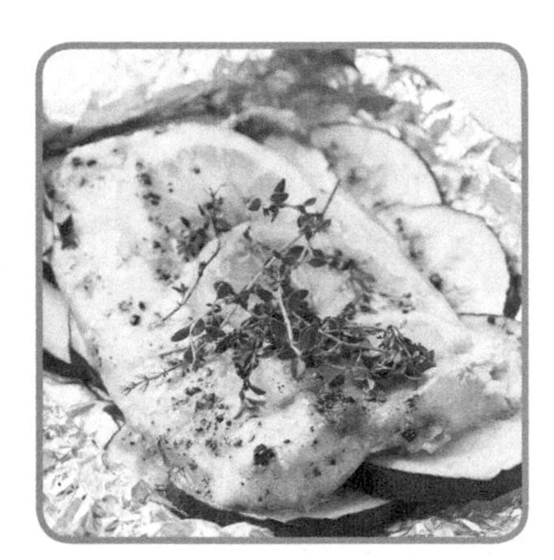

DAY TWO

Breakfast: Salmon & cucumber (see page 85)

Lunch: Asian lettuce wraps (see page 92)

Dinner: Stir-fry on cauliflower (see page 99)

Snack: Soup of choice (see page 105)

Total Calories: 826

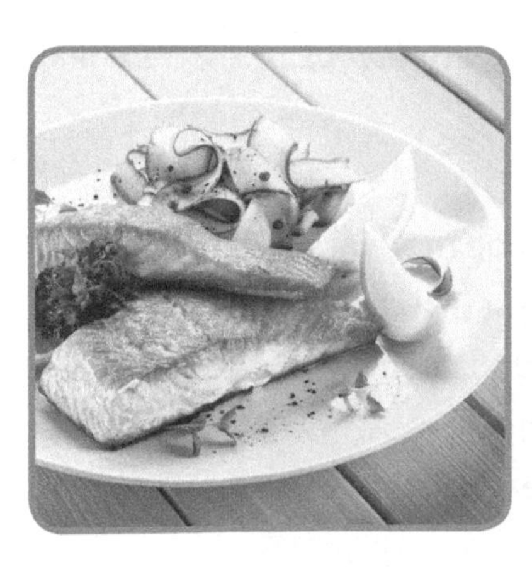

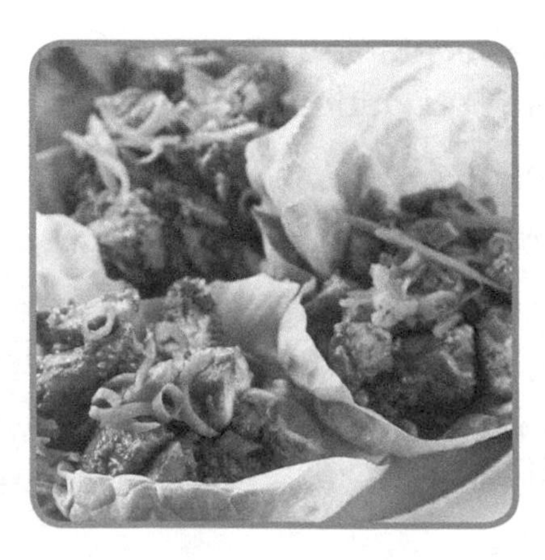

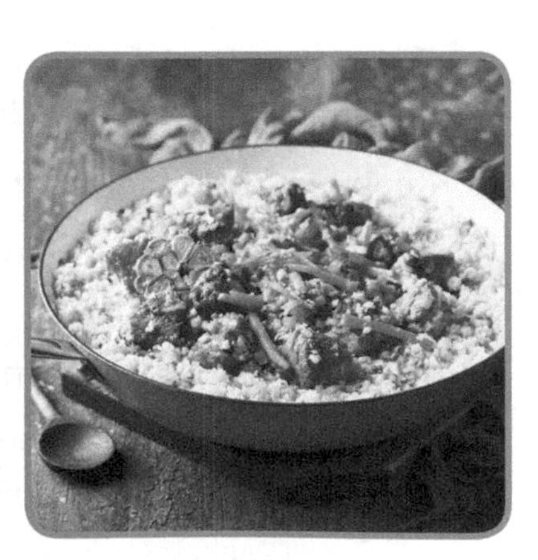

DAY THREE

Breakfast: Rainbow omelet (see page 86)

Lunch: Chicken salad (see page 93)

Dinner: Lettuce burger (see page 100)

Snack: Soup of choice (see page 105)

Total Calories: 826

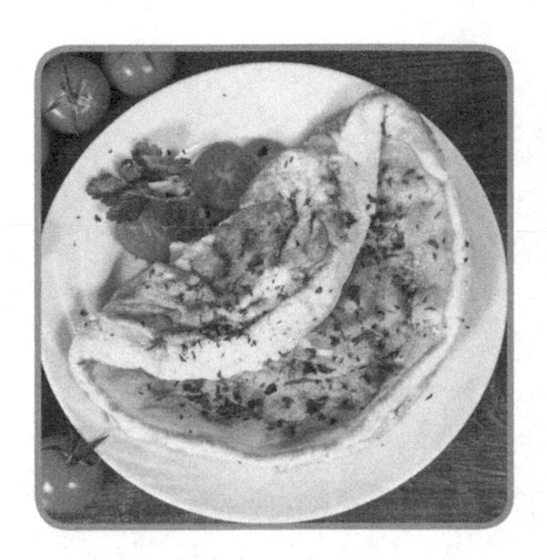

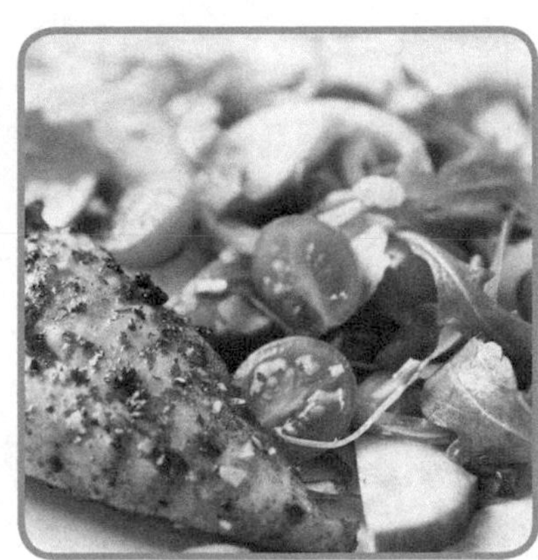

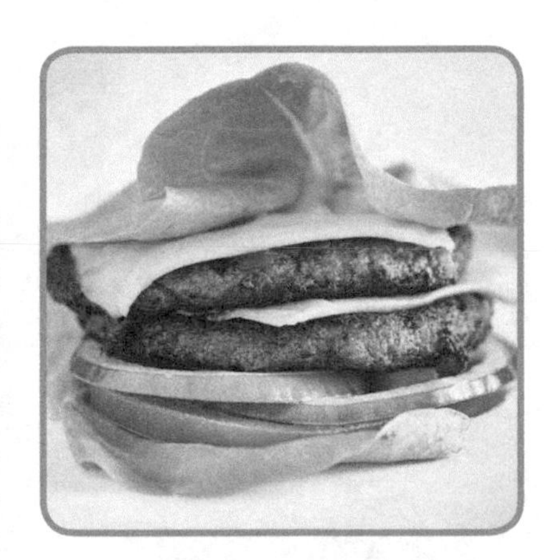

DAY FOUR

Breakfast: Steak & zucchini (see page 87)

Lunch: Zucchini pasta (see page 94)

Dinner: Chicken & cucumber (see page 101)

Snack: Soup of choice (see page 105)

Total Calories: 821

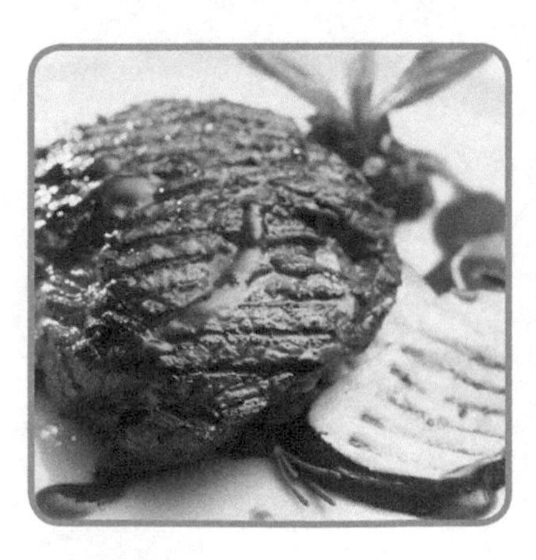

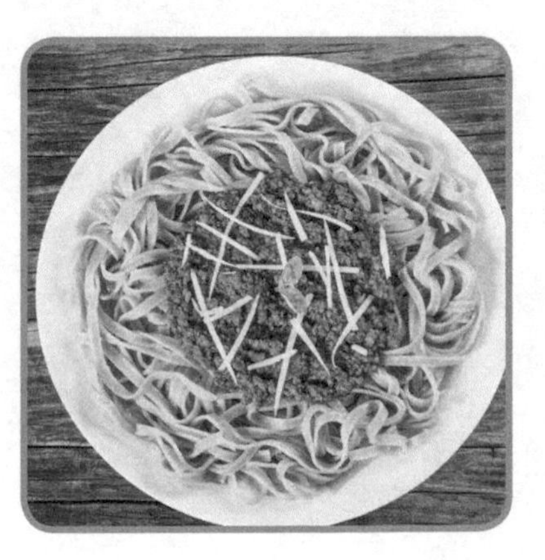

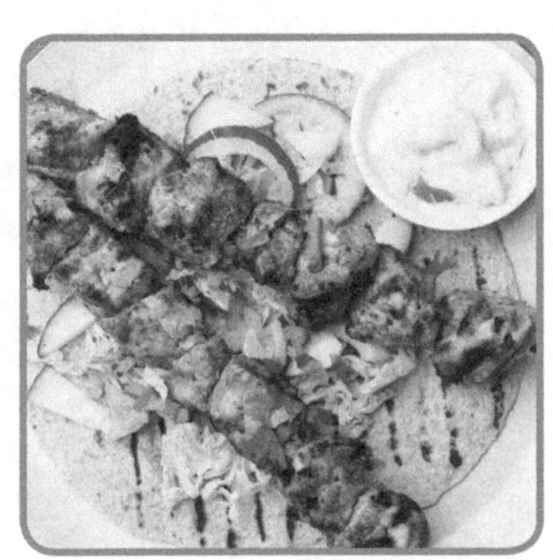

DAY FIVE

Breakfast: Scrambled eggs (see page 88)

Lunch: Shrimp on rice (see page 95)

Dinner: Lamb chops & brussels (see page 102)

Snack: Soup of choice (see page 105)

Total Calories: 801

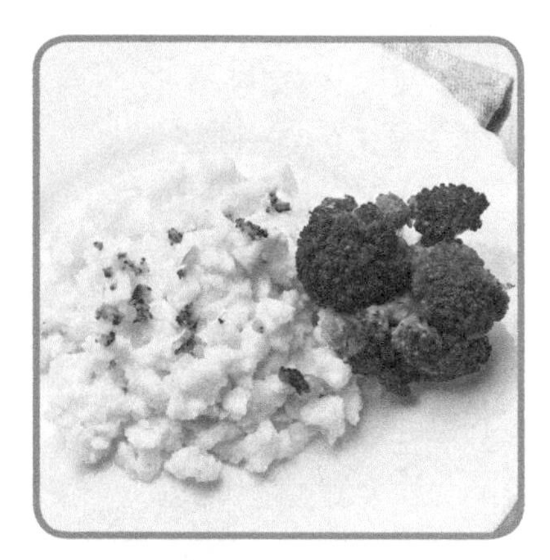

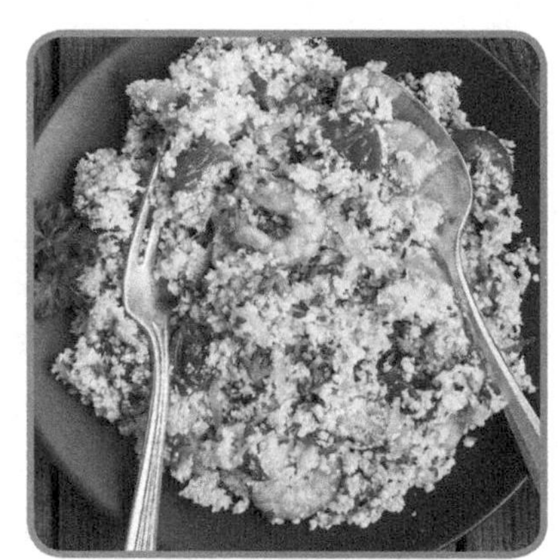

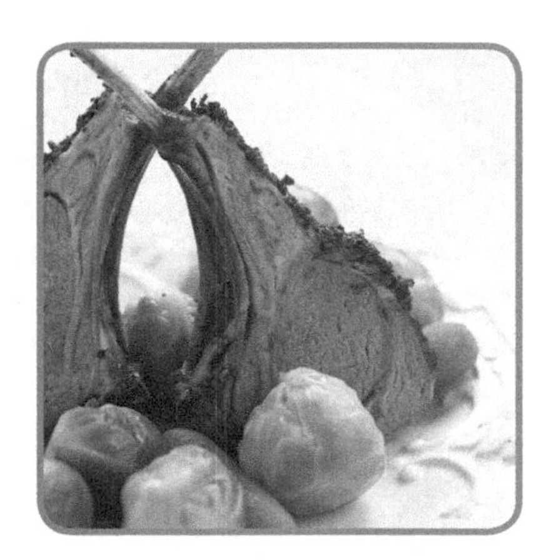

DAY SIX

Breakfast: Egg couscous (see page 89)

Lunch: Pork chops & bok choy (see page 96)

Dinner: Turkey & Cauliflower (see page 103)

Snack: Soup of choice (see page 105)

Total Calories: 821

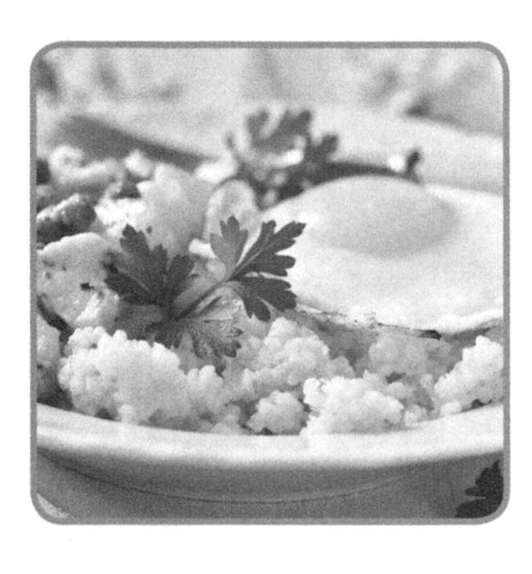

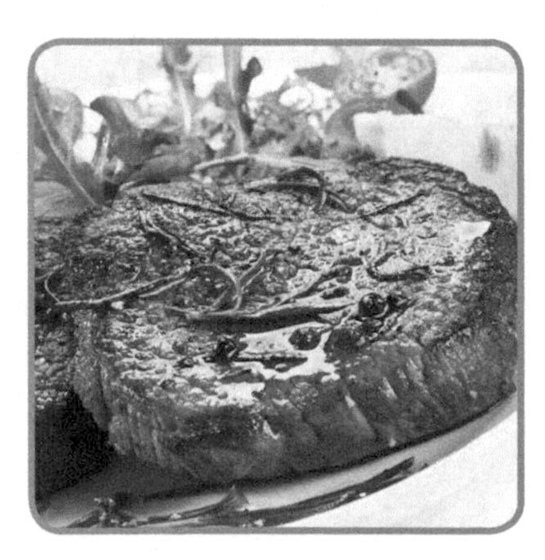

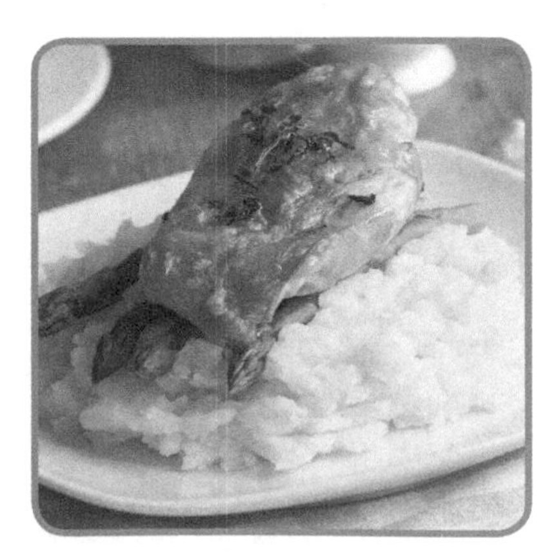

DAY SEVEN

Breakfast: Stuffed mushrooms (see page 90)

Lunch: Turkey wraps (see page 97)

Dinner: Zucchini lasagna (see page 104)

Snack: Soup of choice (see page 105)

Total Calories: 810

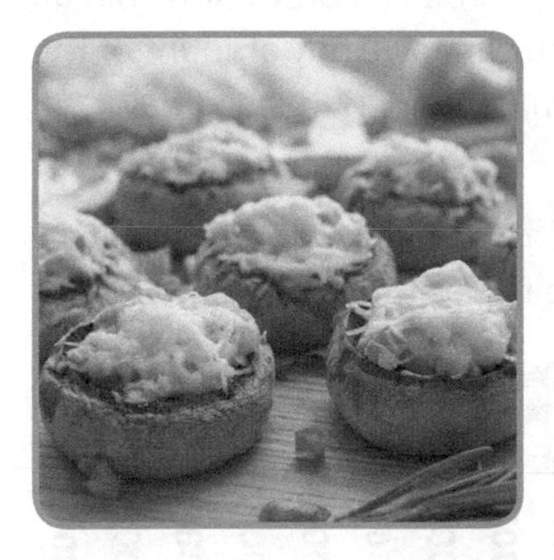

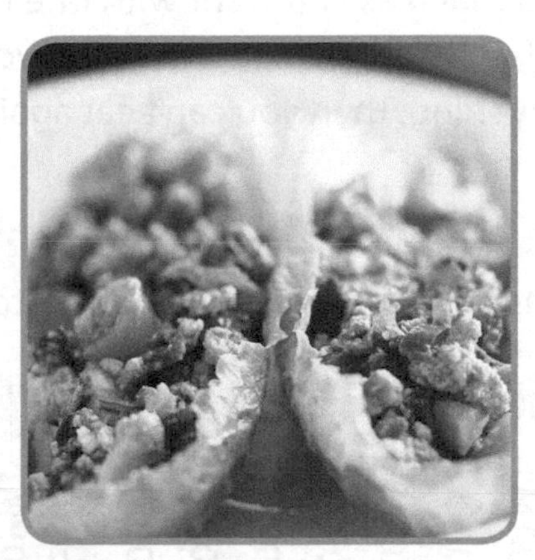

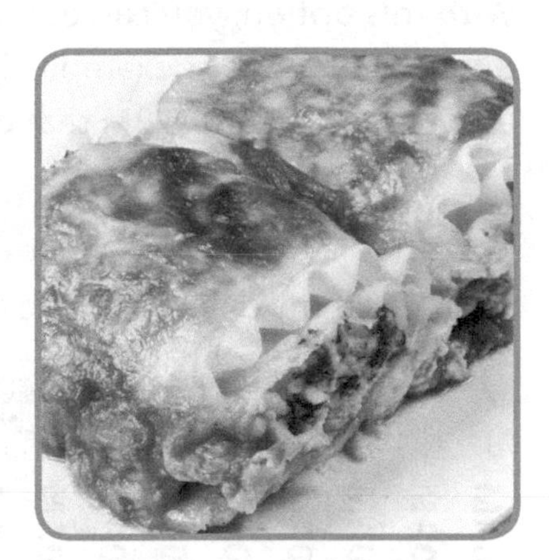

SOUPS - ONE PER DAY

Soup #1: Vegan noodle soup(see page 105)

Soup #2: All-vegetable soup (see page 106)

Soup #3: Tomato soup (see page 107)

Total Calories: 60-75 each

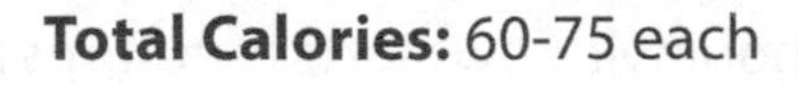

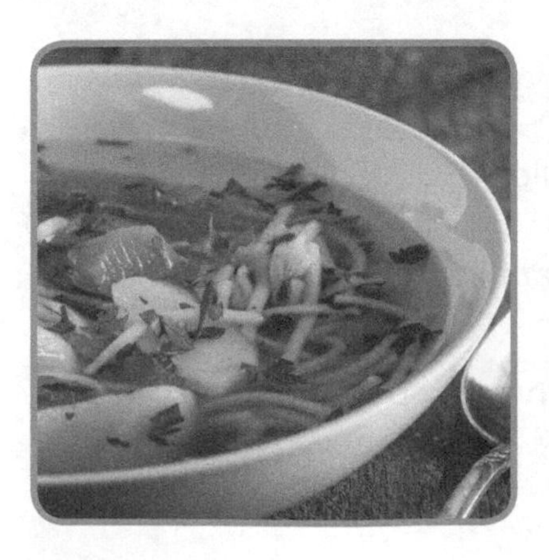

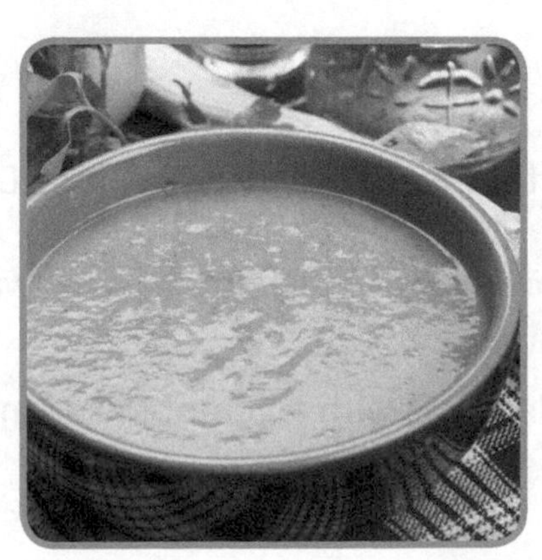

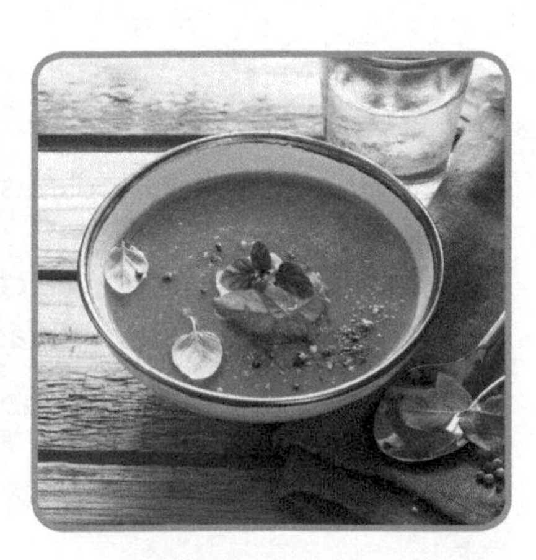

Option 2: Slow & Steady (3-6 Months)

The second option is much easier to follow; it just takes longer. It works on the principles of intermittent fasting. It will still unclog your liver and reverse Type 2 diabetes.

The diet works in conjunction with the Liver Cleansing supplement to complete reverse diabetes as quickly as possible. If you don't already have them, they are available at *www.GetSugarBalance.com/Discount*

Depending on how clogged your liver is, this can take anywhere between 3-6 months to complete.

With this option, you can eat as much as you want with one rule. You can only eat within an 8-hour window. For example, if you had breakfast at noon, you can have any amount of the allowed foods until 8 PM that evening, then you can't eat again until noon the next day.

My 24 Hour 18/6 Intermittent Fasting Time-line

This is my day-to-day life as far as a routine goes. I stick to this as much as possible!

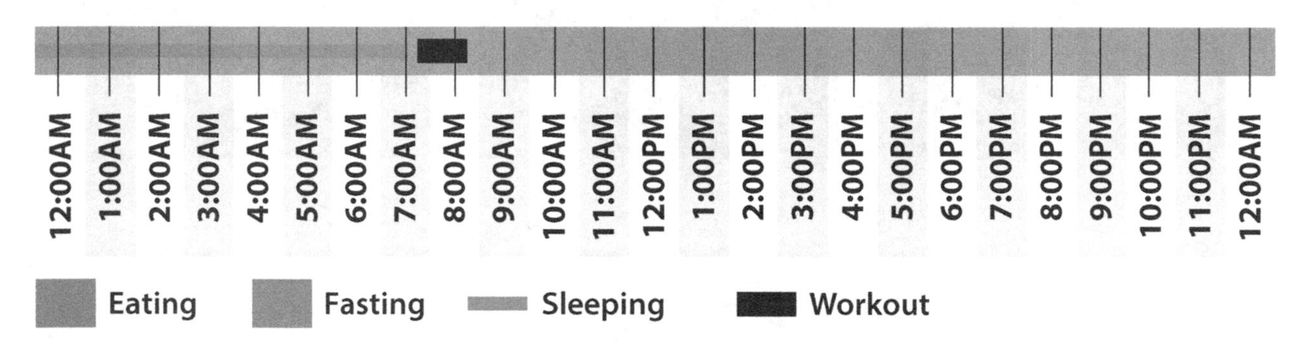

When the 8-hour window starts and stops is up to you. The great part is sleeping is included in the 16-hour fasting time. The only thing you can consume during the fasting period is water and unsweetened tea. You still need to drink at least two liters of water each day. Most people find this option to be the easiest one.

What to Eat & Drink

Here are the simple guidelines for the Slow & Steady Calorie Diet:

- For 3-6 months, you will consume as much food as you want in an 8-hour period, then 16 hours a day of water fasting
- The diet will focus on whole foods with an emphasis on non-starchy vegetables, eggs, seafood, and meat.

- » You must drink at least two liters of pure water per day. If you don't like the flavor, add some fresh-squeezed lemon juice.
- » You can find delicious recipes near the end of this book. Eat any combination you want as long as it's within the 8-hour window. You can use most paleo recipes as long as they only use foods from the list below.

ALLOWED FOODS (YOU CAN EAT ANY OF THE FOODS BELOW.)			
All meat	Cauliflower	Celery	Spinach
All poultry	Asparagus	Tomatoes	Brussel Sprouts
All seafood	Mushrooms	Zucchini	Radishes
Eggs	Kale	Onions	Okra
Peppers	Cucumbers	Eggplant	Fennel
Broccoli	Lettuce	Cabbage	Bok Choy
Herbs: Parsley, cilantro, basil, rosemary, thyme, pepper, garlic Salt: small amounts of sea salt Fat: All oils, lard, ghee, coconut oil, avocados			

Slow & Steady Tips

Here are a few tips to make this option a little easier:

- » Avoid processed foods at all costs. There are often chemicals in the food to make you hungry. Try not to shop on an empty stomach. This will only lead to poor choices.
- » If you get hungry during the fasting portion of the day, drink some unsweetened tea.
- » Keep tempting foods out of the house and out of sight.
- » Weigh yourself often; this will motivate you to keep going.
- » If you must go to a restaurant, tell the waiter you're diabetic and make sure there are no extra sauces or sugar added to the meal. They usually include sugar in meats and salads.

» If you're not sure if a food has sugar in it, use a Diastix stick to measure. Put a small amount of the food in your mouth and mix it with your saliva. Then spit a tiny bit onto a test strip. Any color change indicates the presence of sugar.

» Alcohol should be avoided if possible. If you must have some, limit it to one ounce of vodka, tequila, or whisky, or one cup of dry white wine per day.

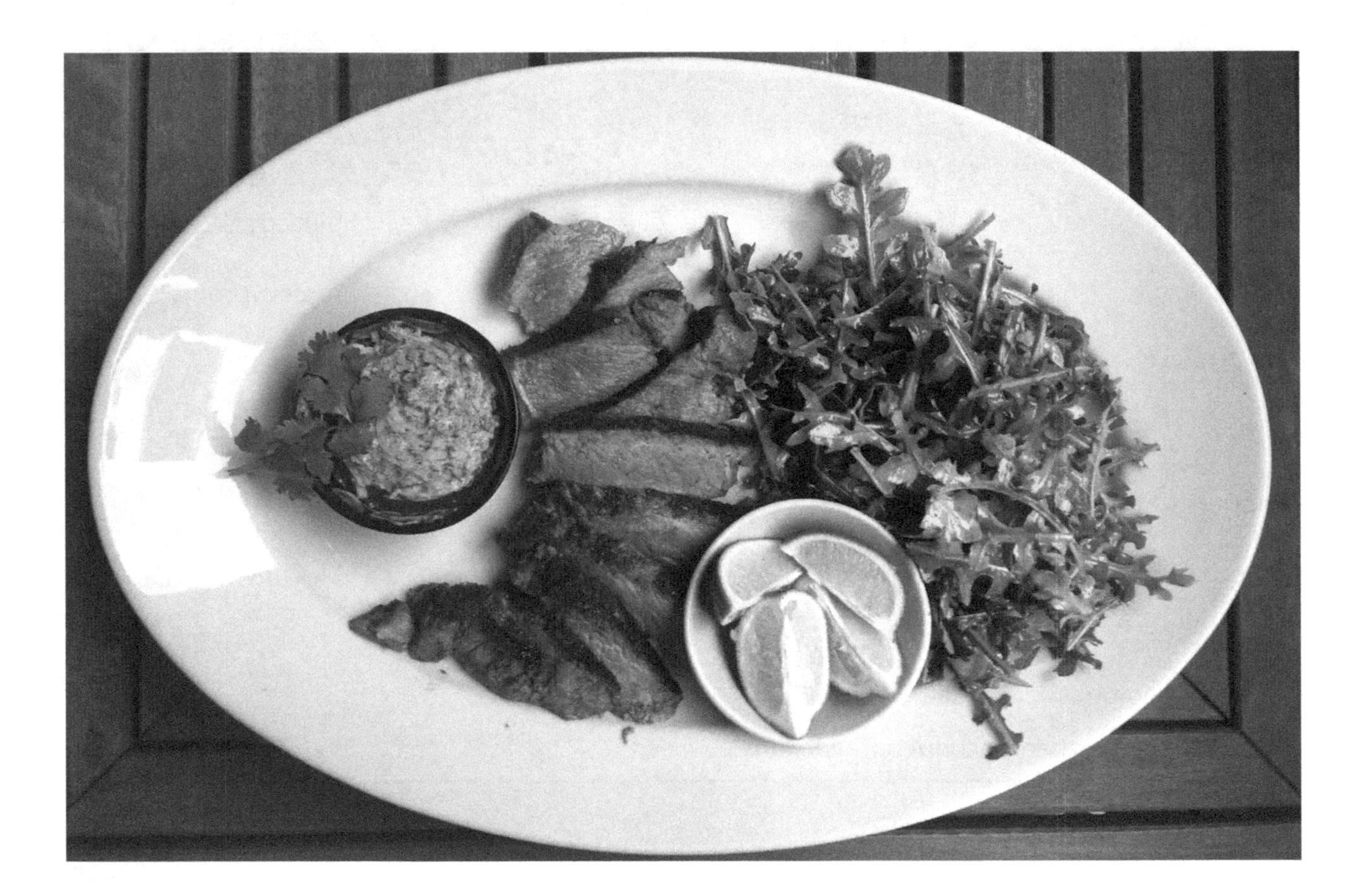

Recap: No-No Foods (Not allowed on either diet)

SWEETS & SWEETENERS

- Artificial sweeteners (other than pure stevia)
- Candies, especially so called sugar-free types
- Honey and fructose
- Foods containing products whose names end in -ol or -ose (dextrose, glucose, lactose, mannitol, mannose, sorbitol, sucrose, xylitol, xylose)
- Also, corn syrup, molasses, agave and maltodextrin.

SWEET OR STARCHY VEGETABLES

- Beans: chili beans, chickpeas, lima beans, lentils, sweet peas, string beans, snow peas.
- Beets
- Carrots
- Corn
- Parsnips
- Potatoes
- Squash & Pumpkins

FRUITS & JUICES

- All fruits
- All juices

DAIRY

- All dairy

GRAINS & GRAIN PRODUCTS

- Wheat, rye barley, corn, oats, and lesser known alternative such as kasha, quinoa, buckwheat and sorghum
- White rice, brown rice, wild rice or rice cakes
- All pasta
- All breakfast cereals
- Pancakes and waffles
- Bread, crackers, and other flour products including whole grain breads

PREPARED FOOD

- Most commercially prepared soups
- Most packaged "health foods"
- Anything in a box, bag or can
- Snack foods including chocolate
- Balsamic vinegar (use wine vinegar, white vinegar, or cider vinegar instead)

How Do You Know When You're Done?

That's easy. Once you've been on the diet for at least 3 months without any medication you can stop and move to the Diabetes Free Forever stage of the program.

Diabetes Free Forever

So ... you've completed the FastTrack or the Slow & Steady diet, and you're diabetes free, so now what?

As you learned earlier in this chapter, the reason you became diabetic in the first place is because you were eating the wrong foods or eating them in the wrong combinations.

Now you *could* ignore everything I'm about to say and eat all the junk you want, but it's only a matter of time before you clog up your liver all over again. This could be years from now or sooner, depending on how badly you eat. You can always repeat the Diabetes Free Program again when that happens, but there's a better way.

All you need to do is follow a few simple rules, and your diabetes will never return. And don't worry – you can still enjoy your favorite foods in moderation.

I don't want to needlessly complicate this, so here are the five simple rules:

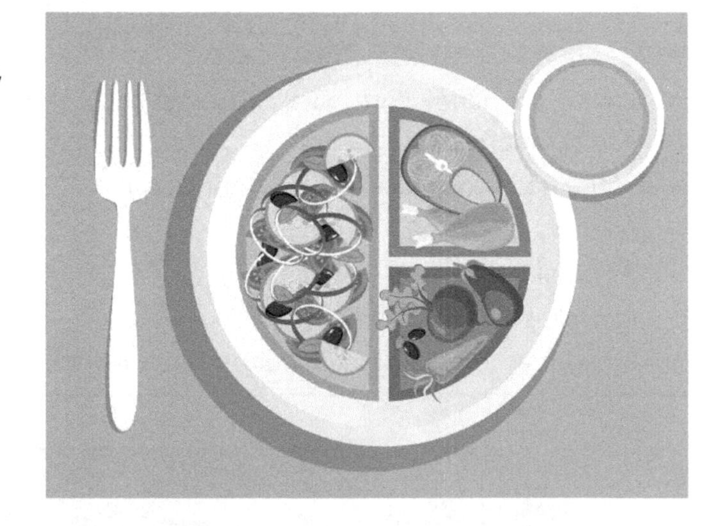

1. For most of your meals, eat a whole foods diet primarily made up of fruit, vegetables, and meat. This means nothing from a box, bag, or can. It's okay to cheat once in a while.
2. Follow the 80/20 principle. For most your meals, make 80% of your plate any combination of vegetables and 20% meat.
3. Completely cut out milk and other dairy products (including cheese).
4. Consider fasting for 16-hours a day on weekends. This will give your liver a chance to clean up any fat you've accumulated during the week.
5. Drink plenty of pure water (I like distilled). Aim for two liters per day. Skip all those sugary drinks.

And that's it. That's all you have to do to stay diabetes free forever. Again, it doesn't matter if you cheat once in a while. What's important is how consistently you eat over time.

You now have everything you need to start the Diabetes Free Program and change your life forever.

I'm going to go over a few more ideas that will accelerate your results.

CHAPTER 7

RECOMMENDED EXERCISES TO ACCELERATE RESULTS

Exercise is vital to your health even if you don't have diabetes. But for those that do, it's particularly important in controlling your blood sugar levels. As I've said before, most Type 2 diabetics naturally produce too much insulin, and the fastest, most effective way to reduce blood sugar levels is to get more exercise.

It even helps accelerate the unclogging of your liver and pancreas which further improves your blood sugar levels.

The problem is, exercise is tedious or unpleasant for most people. In this chapter, I'm going to show you some simple techniques you can use to get the maximum benefits from the minimum amount of time.

Walking for Health

Walking is one of the most rewarding physical activities one can do. Our bodies thrive on walking, especially when we do so outdoors. And unlike other forms of exercise, walking is low impact. This means you're much less likely to get injured or wear out your knees.

Your aim should be about 10,000 steps per day. This is the minimum I recommend to maintain good health and keep weight off. It might be a good idea to get a pedometer to track your steps. You can find high quality ones online for as little as $10. If you keep your mobile phone with you at all time, you can also download an app to track your steps.

If you're like most people, you average around 5,000 steps a day or less, so you're going to have to make a few changes to hit your new target. If you add an additional 500 steps each week you are on the Diabetes Free Program, you should be close to the magic number of 10,000 steps at the end of eight weeks.

Also, it might be time to invest in some comfortable shoes; this is especially true for diabetics who have more foot problems. If you have insurance, consider orthopedic shoes that are made to measure. You may even want to buy special walking soles with extra padding.

The best way to increase your steps is to build more of them into your daily life. Here are some ideas:

- Always take the stairs.
- Always walk when you're on escalators.
- Walk kids to school or the bus stop.
- Walk the dog for an extra block.
- If you take public transportation, get off one stop earlier.
- Park your car at the far end of the parking lot.
- Stand at your desk instead of sitting when at all possible. Visit colleagues in person instead of calling or sending emails.
- Walk on the spot while watching TV or scrolling through Facebook.
- Taking up activates such as gardening or dancing.
- Join a walking group.

Strength Training

As you get older, your muscles can begin to shrink if you don't use them. To keep your muscles strong, you need to add some form of resistance training.

I personally don't like going to the gym. I don't have time to travel there and wait in line to use the machines. Instead, I do a simple regimen that you can do anywhere.

It focuses on all of the major muscle groups in order to have the maximum impact. It's based on research from the American College of Sports Medicine. All you need to do is follow these five exercises, three times per week. They only take a few minutes, and you can do them anytime during the day. Here are the five exercises:

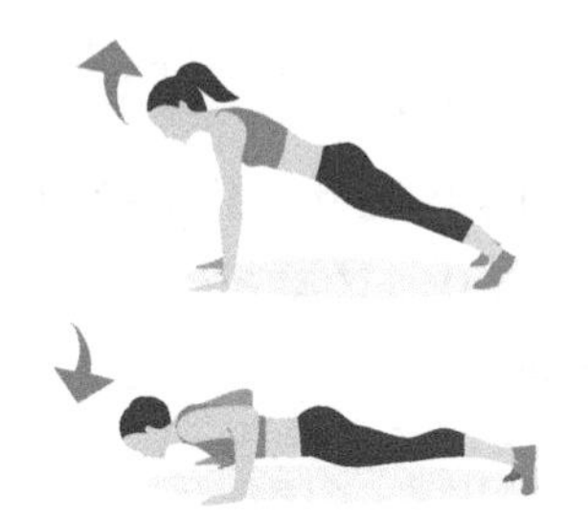

PUSH-UPS
Get into the push-up position with your hands under your shoulders and the balls of your feet touching the ground. Keep your body straight. If it's too hard, do vertical push-ups against a counter or even a wall. Do as many push-ups as you can do within two minutes.

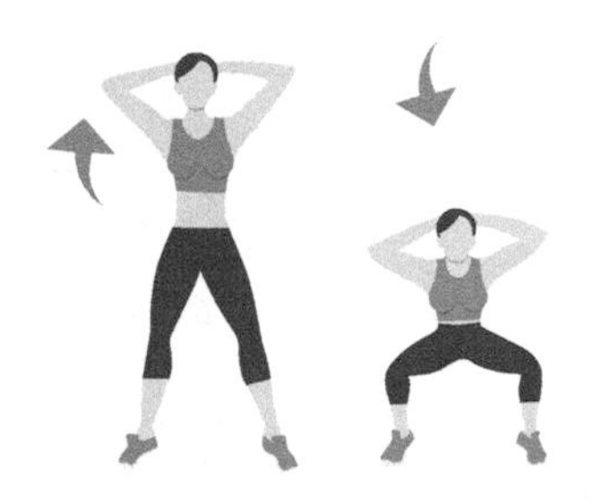

SQUATS
Stand with your feet shoulder width apart. Sit down like you're sitting on an imaginary chair. Remember to keep your back straight. Do as many squats as you can within two minutes while maintaining proper form.

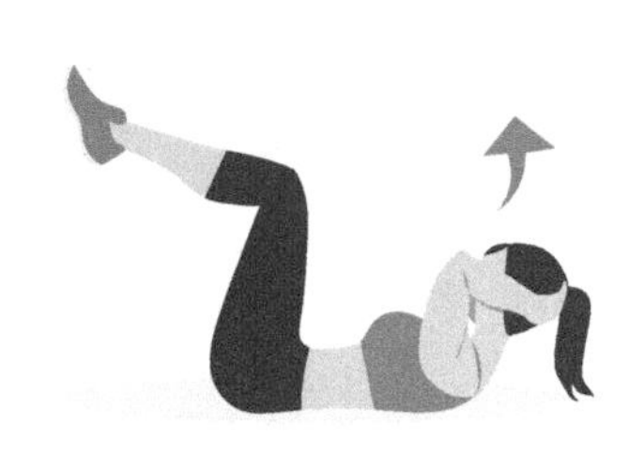

CRUNCHES
Lie on your back with your knees bent and feet flat on the floor. Place your hands on the sides of your head. Gently pull your abdominals inward while curling your head, neck, and shoulder blades off the floor. Do as many crunches as you can within two minutes.

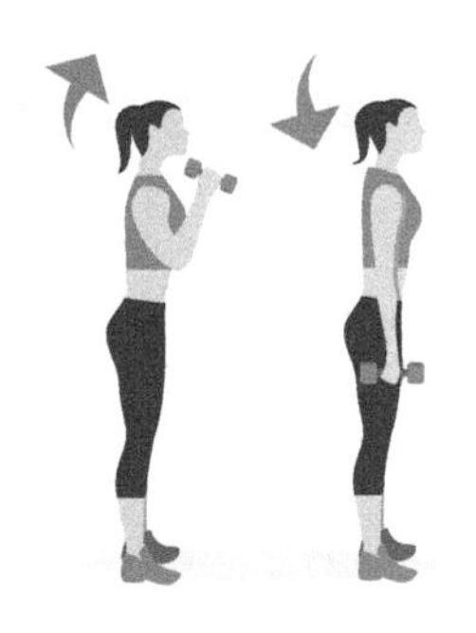

BICEP CURLS
Stand up straight with a dumbbell in each hand. If you don't have dumbbells, pick up anything that has a similar weight. Keeping your upper arms stationary, curl your arms to your shoulders and then lower them. Repeat this as many times as you can within two minutes.

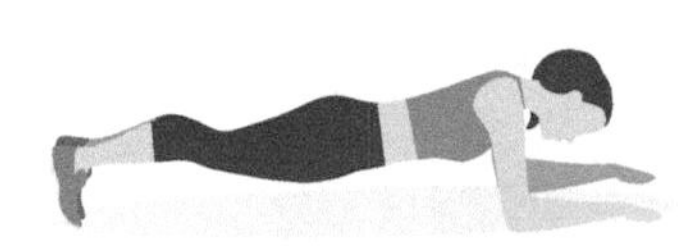

PLANKS
Start by getting into a push-up position. Bend your elbows and rest your weight on your forearms. Your body should form a straight line from shoulders to ankles. Engage your core by sucking your belly button into your spine. Hold this position as long as you can within two minutes.

Getting More Vigorous Activity

The standard recommendation is to do at least 150 minutes of moderate aerobic activity or 75 minutes of vigorous aerobic active each week. Most of us don't come close to this, and the most common excuse I hear is, "I don't have enough time."

This is where a new approach to exercise comes in. It's called High Intensity Interval Training or HIIT. It's a form of interval training alternating between short periods of intense aerobic exercise with less intense recovery periods of exercise.

It's short and intense, and that's why HIIT has become a popular way to burn more fat, improve endurance, and build strength. So the excuse that you don't have the time is no longer allowed, because you can get a great cardio workout in as little as five minutes.

The amount of HIIT programs available could fit a book on their own, so the best way to find something that suits your needs is to search for "HIIT Workout" on the internet. There are many free resources that can give you detailed information about how to perform the exercises.

Whatever you choose, just make an effort to increase your physical activity each and every day. It will not only help your diabetes, but it will also help your overall health as well.

CHAPTER 8

OPTIONAL - HEALING WITH YOUR MIND

In the past decade or so, hundreds of studies have been conducted that demonstrate the **powerful connection between mind and body**. While Napoleon Hill figured it out many years ago, many scientists now believe that what you think about actually shapes your life.

For example, if you truly believe you need insulin injections to balance your blood sugar levels, your body will agree. Research has shown that your body changes the chemicals it makes (including insulin) based on what you're thinking about.

In landmark studies, Dr. Bruce Lipton proved that your mind can affect the cells of your body and even your DNA. It goes on to explain how our expectations and desires can affect our bodies ability to fight illnesses and heal itself.

So how do you use this "natural power" to heal your diabetes? Let's find out.

Is Your Subconscious Keeping You Diabetic?

Each and every one of us has an image of ourselves in our subconscious mind. Your current self-image is built and shaped by the interpretations and evaluations you place on past experiences.

For example, let's just say that at some point of time in your past, someone may have mentioned that diabetes runs in your family. Now regardless of whether you were at a higher risk to get diabetes or not, you may have started thinking that you were. You may have imagined yourself being diabetic. This may be something that you consciously or subconsciously remember and play it out in your mind.

My point is that it doesn't matter if the experience is real or imagined – your mind sees them the same, and these thoughts affect your self-image. Your mind and body react to your internal self-image. So if your self-image is one of a diabetic, your body will do everything it can to make that true.

In order to be diabetes free for life, it's best to change your self-image. Luckily, there's an easy way to do this.

21-Day Visualization Exercises

The mind is a powerful thing to waste. It can do so much for us, and very few of us actually use its power to shape our self-image and create perfect health.

The first thing to do is get a clear image in your mind's eye of what it would feel like to be diabetes free – the ideal you.

Begin by imagining yourself completely free of diabetes ... free of insulin shots and medication ... eating all of the foods you love.

I promise you, if you give this an honest effort, you'll be so thrilled with the results, and you'll choose to continue using this tool for the rest of your life.

We have purposefully asked you to challenge yourself for three weeks, because research has proven that it takes 21 days to make a substantial change of your self-image.

As I've said before, your current self-image was created by your imagination, so we can use this same method to create a new self-image where you enjoy your perfectly healthy body.

Remember – all you have to do is sit back, relax, and imagine yourself as you wish to be. Here's how...

STEP 1

Grab a piece of paper, and write a brief description of the image you intend to view in your mind. This will be the movie you play repeatedly in your mind.

STEP 2

Every day, find a quiet place to relax where you won't be disturbed. Now close your eyes, and begin playing the movie you wrote about in Step 1 in your mind for at least 20 minutes.

For the first seven days, refine your movie to picture your body exactly as you desire it to be. Then, for the remaining 14 days, play this exact movie in your mind over and over again.

TIP

Most people find they get better results if they imagine themselves sitting in a theater and watching themselves as the star character in a movie on the big screen.

It's important to make your mental movie of yourself as vivid and detailed as possible in order to simulate actual experiences. For example, instead of just picturing your body being healthy, imagine yourself excited as the doctor tells you that you're diabetes free. Imagine your pancreas and its cells working properly again. Imagine how you would feel to be diabetes free.

Pay attention to small details. The more detailed you are, the more your subconscious will believe it to be an actual experience. Make sure to use all of your senses.

CHAPTER 9

QUESTIONS & ANSWERS

What Should I Expect on the 8-Week FastTrack Program?

The First Two Weeks

Many will find the first two weeks to be the toughest as you adjust to eating fewer calories. During this time, you will lose a lot of weight quickly. Some of it will be fat, but a lot of it will be water. As your body starts cleansing itself, it uses water to flush out the fat and other toxins.

That's why it's important for you to drink at least two quarts of water each day. Otherwise, you will become constipated and experience flu-like detox symptoms.

Although everyone is different, here is what you should expect in the first two weeks:

» You may be a little tired in the first week, but you'll get a surge of energy by week two as your body clears out some fat and adjusts to your new diet.

» You may lose between 5-20 pounds of weight. Some of it is water, but a lot of it will be fat.

» In the first few days, your fasting glucose levels may drop 30-50%. This is not uncommon. That's why I recommend working with your doctor to come up with a plan to rapidly reduce your medication.

» By around day 10, many people's blood sugar levels will be normal without medication. Yes, this is under the threshold of what they consider diabetic.

» You may see blood sugar levels fluctuate from time to time. This is normal, so don't let it derail you. It takes time to unclog the liver.

After the First Two Weeks

By the end of two weeks, your body should have fully adjusted to the new diet. Your blood sugar levels will most likely have stabilized to non-diabetic levels, and you probably will have eliminated all or at least most of your medications with the help of your doctor.

For most people, now is not the time to quit. Your liver and pancreas are still likely to have a lot of fat that needs to be cleared out. However, for some people, this may not be the right program. Here are some questions to ask yourself:

1. Are you losing weight at a steady pace? (Weight loss may have slowed, but it should still be rapid.)
2. Is your appetite under control? (Most people feel less hungry at this point.)
3. Are your blood sugar levels going up or are they still all over the map?
4. Are you coping emotionally? (It's normal to feel more irritable, but not if you are seriously depressed.)
5. Are you sticking to the diet most of the time?

If you answered no to two or more questions, this might not be the diet for you. Rather than give up, consider switching to the Slow & Steady version of this program.

The reason for this questionnaire is to see how you are doing on the diet. It doesn't help anyone if you give up at this point and say it doesn't work. I'd rather you switch to the easier version of the program, so that you still get the benefits of Diabetes Free.

PRE-DIABETIC OR THE VERY SLIM ONLY

Not everyone needs to complete the full 8 weeks. If you are pre-diabetic or very slim to begin with, two weeks may be enough. If you are pre-diabetic or very slim, you can move to the Diabetes Free Forever Program once your blood sugar has normalized without medication for one full week.

At the End of the 8 Weeks

By the end of the eight weeks, your body will have transformed. Your energy levels will be up, you'll be sleeping better, and you'll feel a real sense of achievement.

At this point, you'll be diabetes free! Your liver and pancreas should be fully cleared out, and you'll no longer need prescription drugs (including insulin).

It's time to celebrate with your friends and family. It's also a good time to visit your doctor to share the good news. Re-do the tests and see the results for yourself. Not only will your diabetes be clinically reversed, you'll also see a major improvement in every area of your health.

You might even have to go buy some new clothes to match the new, slimmer you. It's also a good time to pull out the photos you took at the beginning of this journey. Take a new photo and post the before and after on Facebook and other social media sites.

Don't forget to send us your testimonial so we can give other diabetics the confidence to try the Diabetes Free Program.

You can add your testimonial by visiting *www.GoDiabetesFree.com/Testimonial*

Actual Results

> *"The changes I've instituted with The Diabetes Free program has brought my blood sugars down to the 80's, numbers I haven't seen in 15 years! Yeah!!"*
>
> DIABETES FREE SUCCESS STORY – CLAUDIA PRICE

What Should I Expect on the Slow & Steady Program?

For some people, going on a low-calorie diet for eight weeks just isn't for them, and that's why we created the Slow & Steady Program. If you selected this option, here's what to expect:

» You won't lose weight as fast as you would with the FastTrack Program, but it should be more effective than conventional dieting.

» Your blood sugar will reduce steadily over the course of the program. How quickly it will drop depends on a lot of factors including your daily calorie consumption, how strictly you follow the diet, and how severe your diabetes is.
» You'll still need to reduce your medication – just not as quickly as in the FastTrack Program. Again, work with your doctor to do this safely.

From what I have seen in the past, this is how long you should expect to be on the Slow & Steady Program to reverse your diabetes:

CURRENT HEALTH	RECOMMEND TREATMENT DURATION
Pre-diabetic or Diabetic for Less than 3 Years	3 Months
Diabetic for 3+ Years or Currently on Insulin	3-6 Months

What If My Blood Sugar Doesn't Improve?

If you are one of the few people who don't experience incredible results with the Diabetes Free Program, don't give up hope.

In most cases, there are three reasons why you didn't get the results you expected:

1. You didn't follow the program properly.
   Although I've done my best to make this information as clear as possible, some of it can still be confusing. Please re-read the entire book cover-to-cover to see if you have missed something. If something still isn't clear or you have a question, don't hesitate to contact our support team at *support@GoDiabetesFree.com*.

2. You're not actually Type 2 diabetic.
   Although this isn't very common, there is a small chance that you have been misdiagnosed. This means instead of having Type 2 diabetes, you may in fact have Type 1. If you aren't getting the results I've promised with this program, I suggest you get your blood sugar and insulin levels re-tested to ensure you are a Type 2 diabetic.

3. There is a blockage preventing your liver from cleansing.
   If you feel you've followed the program properly and are certain that you are a Type 2 diabetic, then your liver is most likely blocked. This means there is a blockage preventing fat from clearing out of your liver.

To remove the blockage, you'll have to perform a Liver Flush. This is a simple, one-day cleanse that expands liver ducts and flushes out large, hardened blockages. To get more information about how to do the cleanse, please visit the member's area or contact customer service.

What Do I Do After I'm Diabetes Free?

Getting this far is a real achievement, but you don't want to undo all the good work by going back to living the way you used to live. It's time to move to the Diabetes Free Forever part of the program.

In the Diabetes Free Forever Program, you'll eat a mostly paleo-style diet. This means lots of vegetables, fats, and animal products.

You'll still be able to eat the junk and sweets you love. Just remember – the more junk you eat, the more likely it will be that you will become diabetic again.

In the gastric bypass study, patients were tested 14 years later, and 83% of them were still diabetes free. This is without being put on a specific diet; these people ate anything they wanted over the course of those 14 years.

This doesn't mean you'll get the same results. It all depends on your body. Eating junk food could cause you to become diabetic a year from now or 10 years from now. Instead, if you choose to closely follow the Diabetes Free Forever Program, your chances of getting diabetes again are virtually zero.

CONCLUSION

You now have everything you need to reverse your diabetes!

This includes the exact 3-Step Plan that has been used by thousands of people to clear out their fatty organs and lower their blood sugar for good. Here's a recap:

Cleanse Your Liver & Pancreas

The proper functioning of your liver and pancreas is crucial to reversing diabetes. In this first step, you'll use a powerful combination of herbs to gentle cleanse and reactivate the cells your organs. *www.GetSugarBalance.com/Discount*

The Diabetes Free Diet

The Diabetes Free Diet is simple. We've broken down the diet into easy-to-understand guidelines, so you can't go wrong. You'll get a choice of two diets – a FastTrack version and one for those who prefer to go Slow & Steady.

Recommended Exercise

For diabetics who want to accelerate their results, adding some light exercising such as walking is a great idea. Exercise helps burn up excess sugar and clear out deposits of fat from the liver and pancreas.

I've made everything as easy as possible, so there's no reason to delay starting right away. We even have a support team to answer any questions you may have.

But the choice on whether or not you have diabetes is now yours. I've given you all the information, but you still have to follow it to see the results for yourself.

I guarantee you'll be shocked by your transformation like so many before you who have used this program.

The time to change your life is now. Don't wait! The devastating effects of diabetes are waiting for you, so do it now. Don't wait another minute.

Join my cause. No one should have to suffer with this terrible disease when there is a simple and effective solution that's proven to work.

I know that once you're diabetes free, you'll want to shout it from the rooftops, so send us your testimonial and help show other diabetes sufferers what's possible.

You can add your testimonial by visiting: *www.GoDiabetesFree.com/Testimonial*.

I can't wait to hear from you. Thank you for taking a chance on Diabetes Free and believing in the Truth. Remember to stay positive, and enjoy your diabetes-free life!

PART 4

DIABETES RECIPES

CHAPTER 11

RECIPES

It's always easier to stick to a new eating plan when your meals are more satisfying. That's why I've created some delicious recipes that are filling and easy to make.

To make it as easy as possible, I've given you two options for the fast – a quick and intense 8-week fast and a slower, easier-to-follow, 3-6 month fast. You choose what's best for you. Let's quickly recap your options:

Option 1: FastTrack - 800 Calorie/Day (8 Weeks)

The first option is the fastest way to unclog your liver and reverse Type 2 diabetes.

For eight short weeks, you eat 800 calories of food each day and drink plenty of water. That might seem low, but it's not as hard as it sounds. Your body will quickly adjust within days, and you'll no longer feel hungry.

You'll find a full, 7-Day meal plan under the FastTrack section below.

Option 2: Slow & Steady (3-6 Months)

The second option is much easier to follow – it just takes longer. It works on the principles of intermittent fasting. It will still unclog your liver and reverse Type 2 diabetes.

Depending on how clogged your liver is, it could take anywhere between 3-6 months to complete.

With this option, you can eat as much of the approved foods as you want with one rule. You can only eat that food within an 8-hour window. For example, if you have breakfast at noon, you can have any amount of the allowed foods until 8 PM that evening, and then you can't eat again until noon the next day.

You'll find a full, 7-Day meal plan under the Slow & Steady section. It's best to eat a big salad and one of the meat recipes with each meal following the 80/20 principle.

For more information on exactly how to follow the diet, please refer to the diet section earlier in this book. I hope you enjoy these recipes on your way to becoming diabetes free.

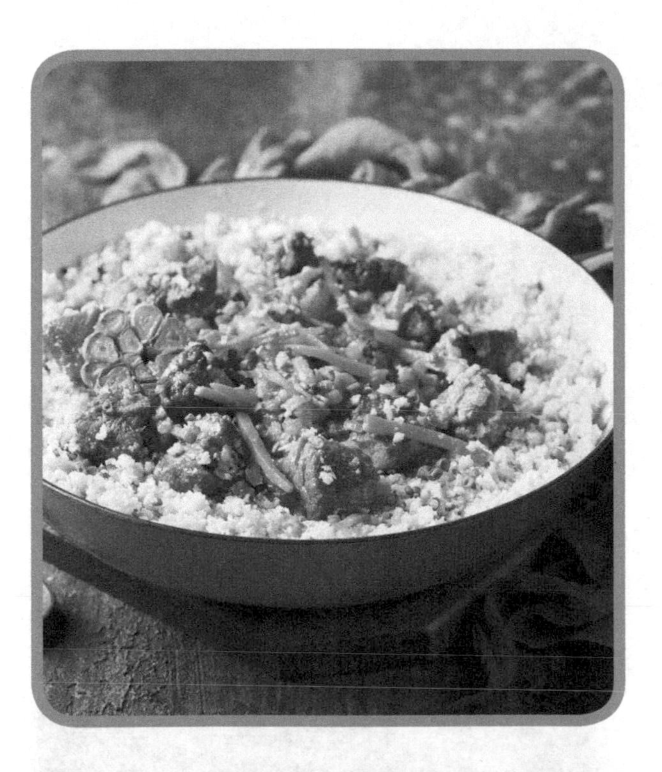

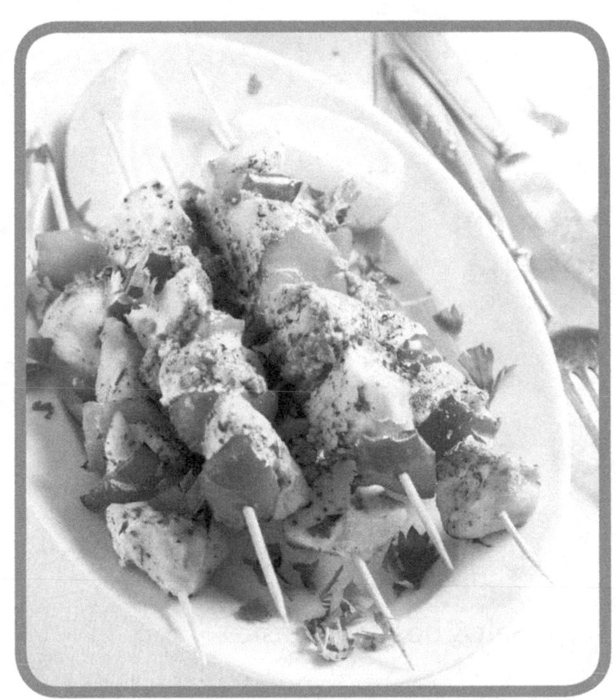

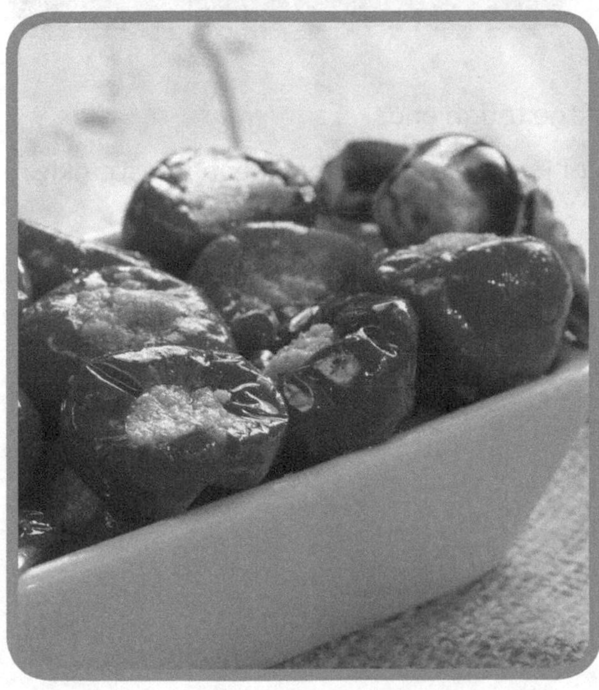

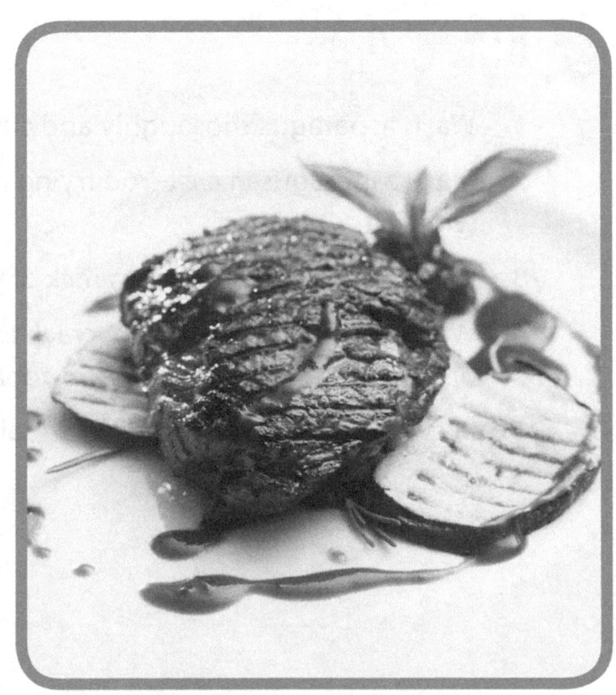

FastTrack

FastTrack Breakfasts

Sunny Side Asparagus

PREP TIME	COOK TIME	CALORIES
5 Min	10 Min	237

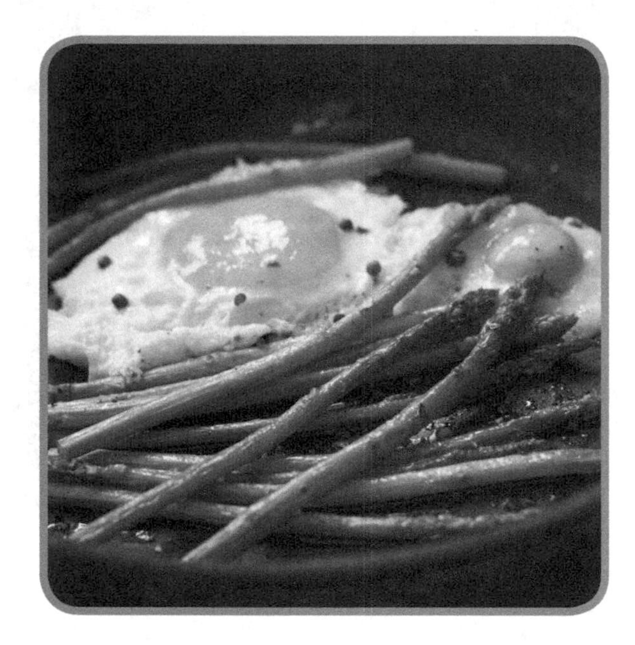

INGREDIENTS

2 large eggs (preferably organic)

3 cups asparagus

Salt & pepper to taste

DIRECTIONS

1. Wash asparagus thoroughly and cut off the tough ends.
2. Place asparagus in cast-iron frying pan or Pyrex glass cooking sheet and sprinkle with salt.
3. Roast asparagus on the top rack of your oven at 450°F for 7-10 minutes.
4. While asparagus is cooking, crack two eggs into a non-stick frying pan and cook on medium heat until eggs are cooked.
5. Serve on plate and sprinkle with salt and pepper to taste.

Savory Salmon & Cucumber

PREP TIME	COOK TIME	CALORIES
10 Min	**15 Min**	**248**

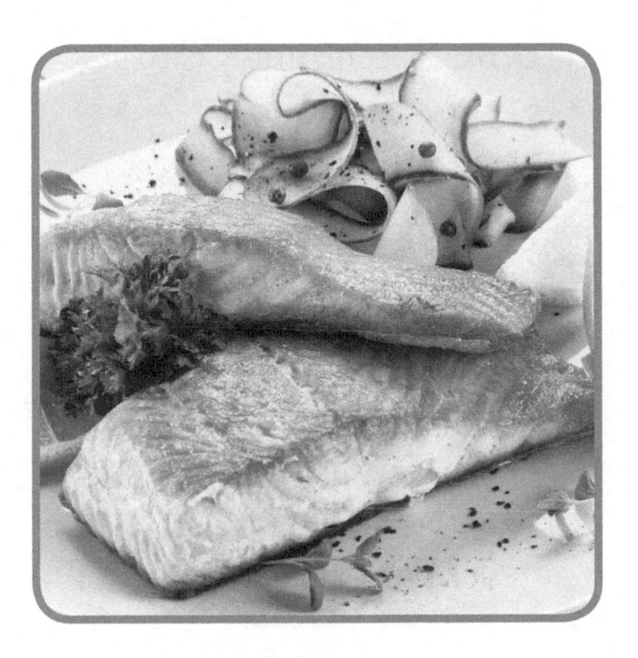

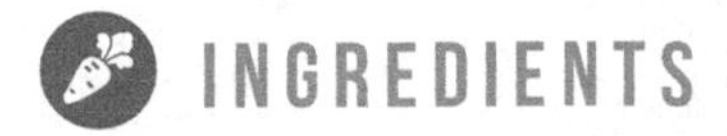

INGREDIENTS

100g salmon filet (preferably ocean caught)

3 cups of sliced cucumbers

2 tablespoons white or apple cider vinegar

1 teaspoon chopped dill

Salt and pepper to taste

DIRECTIONS

1. Preheat oven to 450°F.
2. Season salmon with salt and pepper. Place skin side down on a non-stick baking sheet or pan with ovenproof handle.
3. Bake until salmon is cooked through, about 12-15 minutes.
4. While salmon is cooking, chop cucumber and place in mixing boil.
5. Sprinkle with salt, chopped dill, and vinegar, and mix thoroughly.
6. Serve on plate and enjoy.

Rainbow Omelet & Tomato

PREP TIME	COOK TIME	CALORIES
10 Min	**10 Min**	**245**

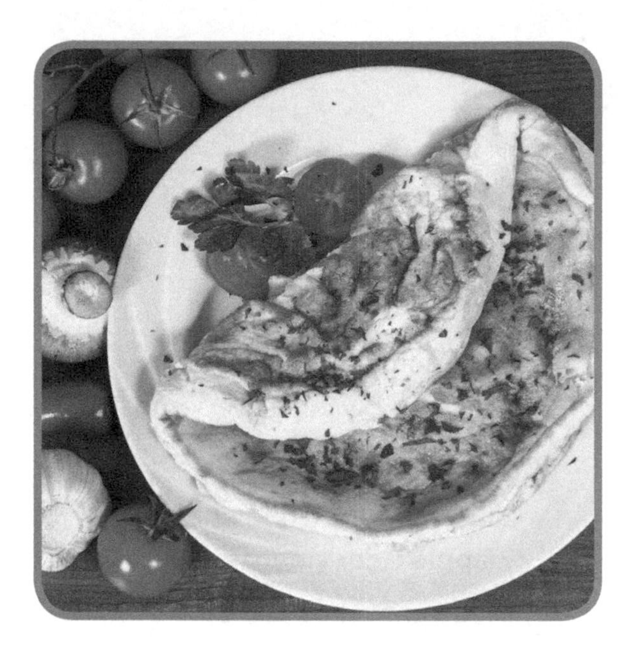

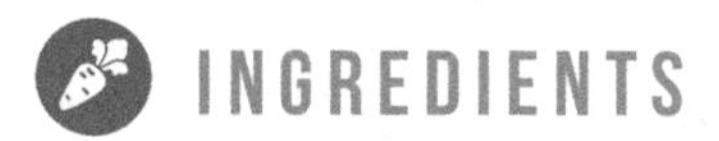

INGREDIENTS

2 large eggs (preferably organic)

2 large tomatoes

2 cup spinach

1 red pepper

Salt & pepper to taste

DIRECTIONS

1. Beat eggs, water, salt, and pepper in a small bowl until blended.
2. Chop spinach and red pepper into fine pieces. Mix into egg.
3. Pour egg mixture into non-stick frying pan and cook over medium heat.
4. While eggs are cooking, slice and salt tomatoes.
5. Once eggs are thoroughly cooked, fold in half to make an omelet.

Sizzling Steak & Zucchini

PREP TIME	COOK TIME	CALORIES
5 Min	15 Min	255

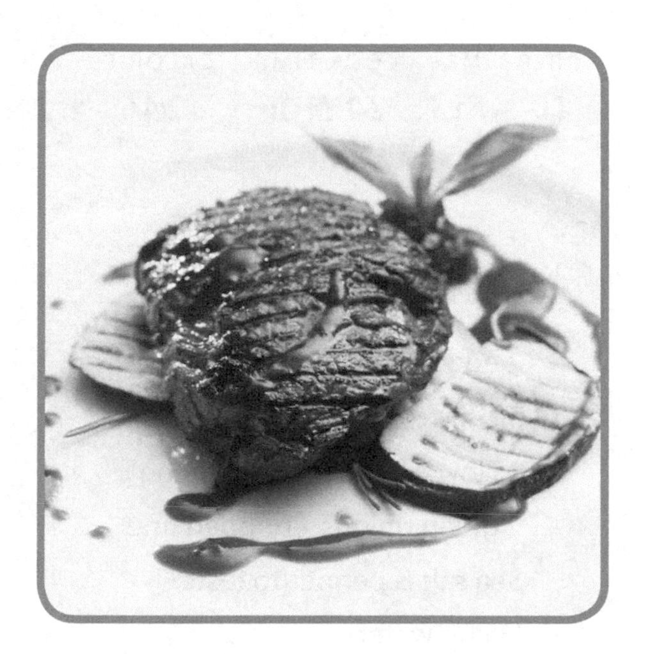

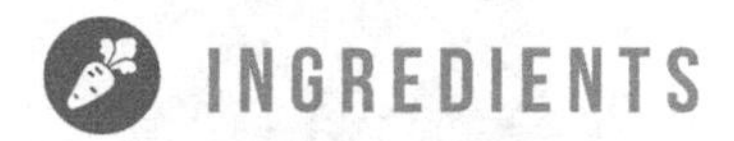

175g lean strip steak
(preferably grass-fed)

3 cups zucchini

Salt & pepper to taste

1 tsp. fresh thyme, chopped

1 tsp. fresh oregano, chopped

1 tsp. fresh parsley, chopped

DIRECTIONS

1. Wash zucchini, cut off the ends, and slice into pieces.
2. Place zucchini in cast-iron frying pan or Pyrex glass cooking sheet and sprinkle with salt.
3. Roast zucchini on the top rack of your oven at 450°F for 7-10 minutes. Also, pre-heat non-stick pan on the stovetop set at medium to medium-high heat for 5 minutes.
4. Season strip steak with salt and pepper.
5. Place steak on heated frying pan, moving the pan around quickly so it doesn't stick. Wait until seared and flip.
6. Once both sides of the steak are browned, place pan in oven for 5 minutes with zucchini.
7. Serve on plate and enjoy.

Scrambled Eggs & Broccoli

PREP TIME	COOK TIME	CALORIES
10 Min	**20 Min**	**246**

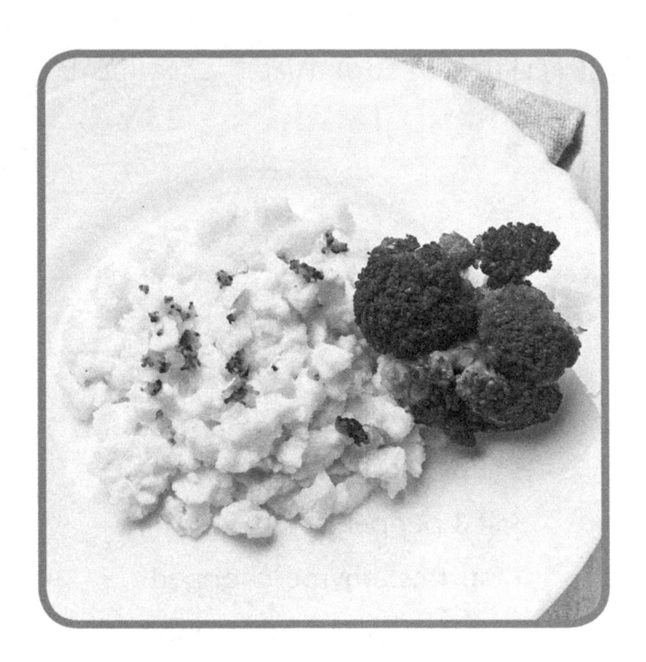

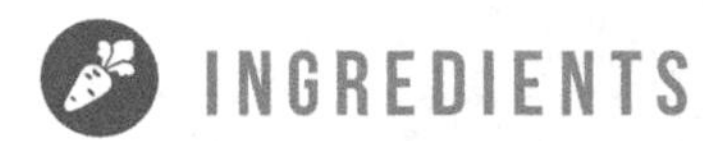

INGREDIENTS

2 eggs (preferably organic)

3 cups of broccoli, chopped fine

2 cloves garlic, chopped fine

2 green onions, chopped fine

Sea salt & pepper to taste

½ cup water

DIRECTIONS

1. In a medium-size, non-stick skillet, add chopped garlic and green onions with enough water to keep them from sticking.
2. Add chopped broccoli, the rest of the water, and sea salt to taste. Let cook for 2-5 minutes or until soft.
3. Add two eggs and gently move the pan around over the heat until fully cooked.

Egg & Cauliflower Couscous

PREP TIME	COOK TIME	CALORIES
10 Min	**10 Min**	**243**

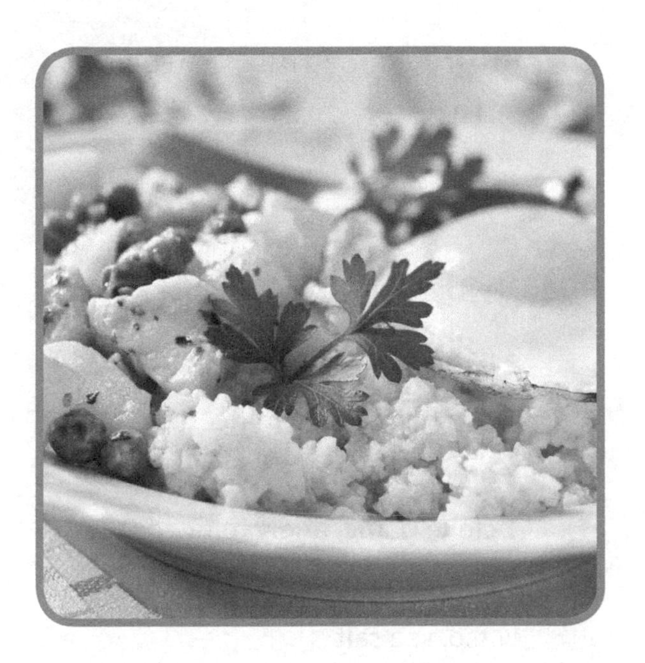

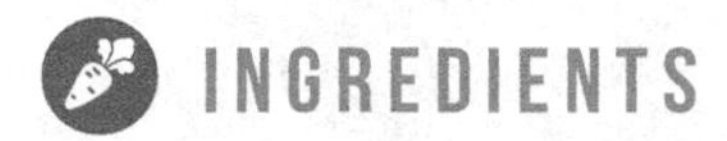

INGREDIENTS

2 large eggs (preferably organic)

3 cups cauliflower

¼ tsp. curry powder, optional

2 green onions, finely chopped

Water

Salt

DIRECTIONS

1. Wash and cut the cauliflower into large pieces.
2. Transfer the cauliflower to a food processor and pulse until completely broken down. It should be processed until it looks like pieces of rice.
3. In a non-stick frying pan over medium heat, add water, processed cauliflower, chopped onions, curry powder, and a pinch of salt. Mix thoroughly and let cook for 3-5 minutes.
4. Place eggs in a pan of cold water, covering the eggs by an inch.
5. Set the pan over high heat and bring the water to a full, rolling boil uncovered.
6. Remove pan from heat and cover. Let sit for 4 minutes.
7. Transfer eggs into a bowl of ice water for 1 minute to peel easier.
8. Serve cauliflower on a plate with soft-boiled eggs on top.

Ham Stuffed Mushrooms

PREP TIME	COOK TIME	CALORIES
10 Min	1 Hour	220

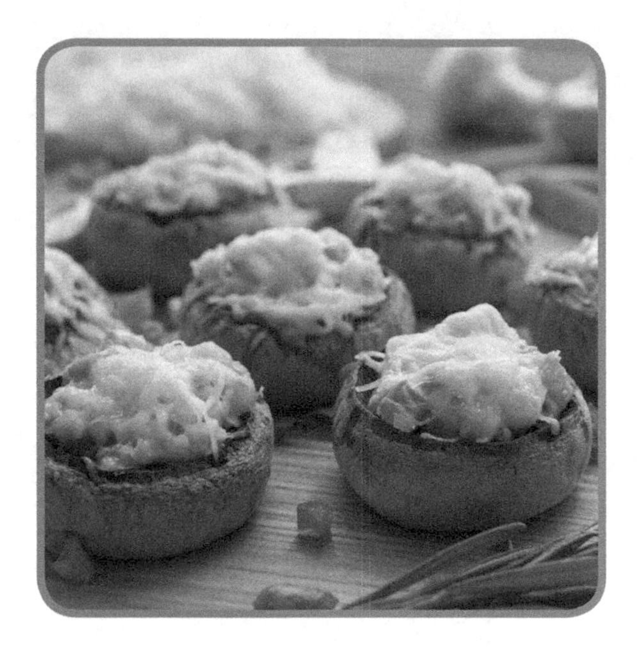

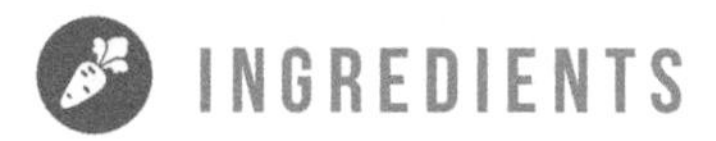

INGREDIENTS

8 large mushrooms

1 cup ham, finely minced

2 green onions

1 clove garlic, finely minced

2 cup baby spinach, chopped

¼ tsp. sea salt

½ tsp. black pepper

Water

DIRECTIONS

1. Wash and trim the end of the stems from mushrooms. Pop remaining stem out. Chop stems and set aside.
2. In a non-stick skillet over medium heat, add chopped onions, garlic, ham, and enough water to keep them from sticking to the pan.
3. Once ham is browned, add baby spinach, salt, and pepper.
4. Preheat oven to 350°F.
5. Place mushroom caps in Pyrex glass cooking sheet, open side up.
6. Fill each cap with a little of the ham stuffing, mounding the filling.
7. Bake for 20 minutes.

FastTrack Lunches

Tuna Stuffed Red Peppers

PREP TIME	COOK TIME	CALORIES
5 Min	**15 Min**	**255**

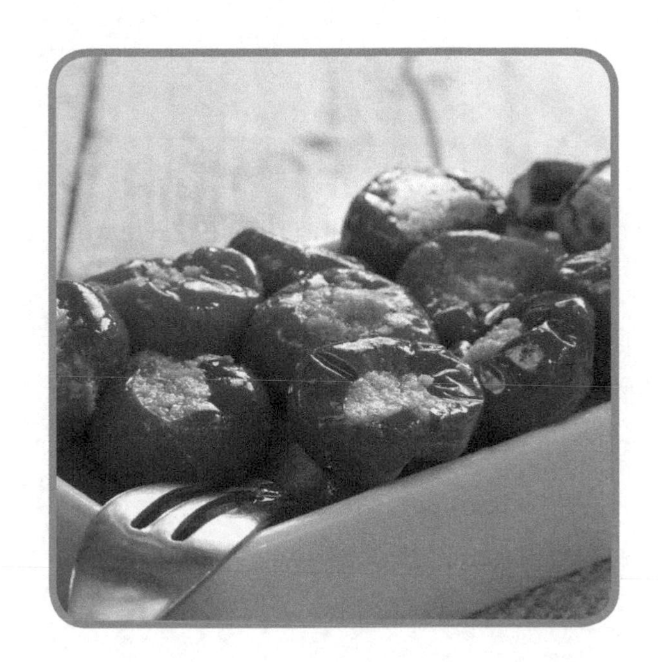

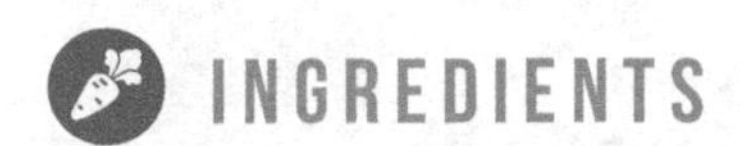

INGREDIENTS

2 large red peppers

1-5 oz. can of light tuna (in water)

½ yellow onion

½ dill weed

½ lemon

Sea salt & pepper to taste

DIRECTIONS

1. Preheat oven to 350°F.
2. Cut two large red peppers in half. With a sharp knife or spoon, carefully remove the inside of the peppers including the seeds.
3. Drain tuna and combine with chopped onions, squeezed lemon juice, dill, and salt & pepper to taste.
4. Stuff into red pepper halves.
5. Place in non-stick Pyrex glass cooking sheet and bake for 15 minutes.

Asian Lettuce Wraps

PREP TIME	COOK TIME	CALORIES
10 Min	15 Min	244

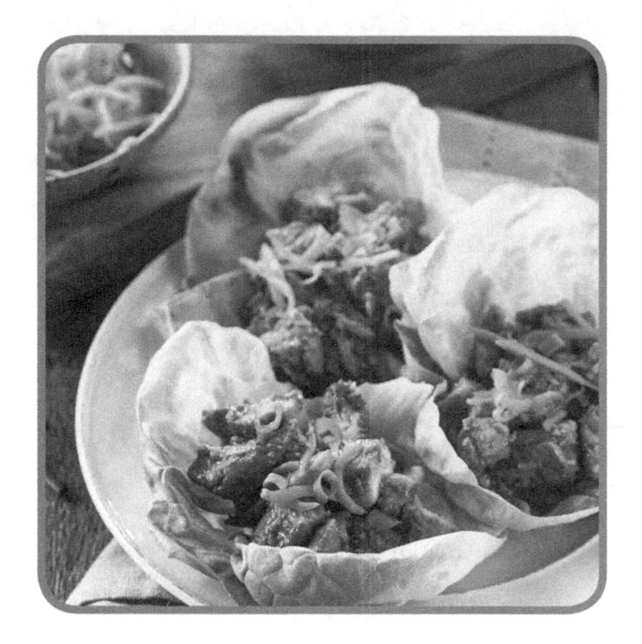

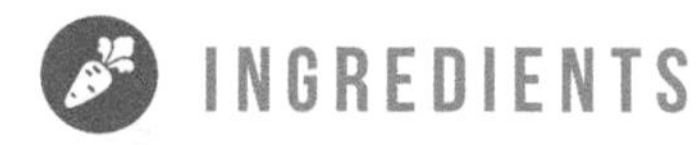

INGREDIENTS

100g lean ground beef (95% lean)

1 yellow onion, chopped

1 green onion stalk

1 red pepper

4 cloves of garlic, diced

6 tbsp. soy sauce

4 large lettuce leaves

DIRECTIONS

1. In a large non-stick pan, add chopped yellow onion, garlic, red pepper, green onion, and water. Keep adding water as needed and cook until soft.
2. Add ground beef and break apart with a cooking spoon. Cook until no longer pink.
3. Add soy sauce and cook everything for a few minutes.
4. To serve, place the meat mixture in the lettuce cups and wrap everything up.

Grilled Chicken Salad

PREP TIME	COOK TIME	CALORIES
15 Min	**5 Min**	**265**

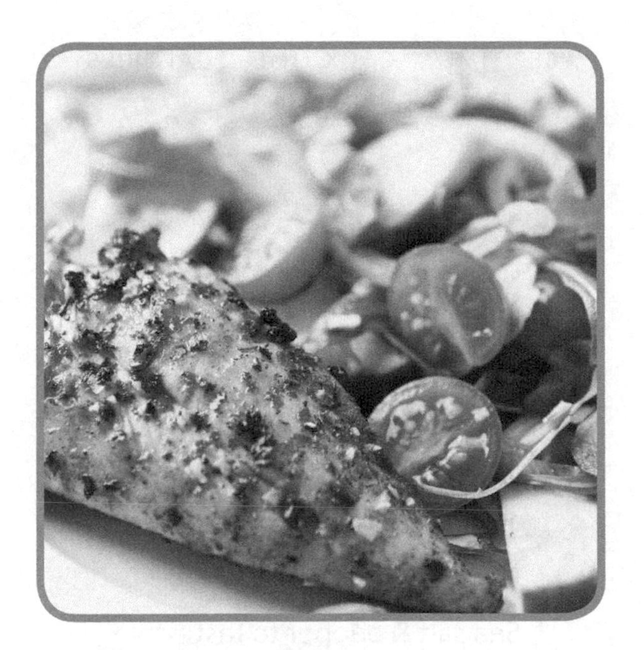

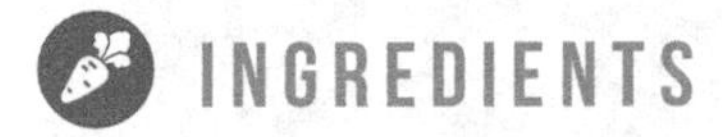

INGREDIENTS

100g lean chicken breast

6 cups chopped cucumbers

2 cups chopped cherry tomatoes

1 garlic clove, finely minced

1 tbsp. chopped dill

3 tbsp. vinegar or fresh lemon juice

Sea salt & pepper to taste

DIRECTIONS

1. Finely mince garlic and add to a small bowl along with vinegar, dill, salt and pepper.
2. Add in chopped tomatoes and cucumbers. Mix thoroughly.
3. Preheat a non-stick skillet to medium high.
4. Season chicken with salt and pepper.
5. Grill the chicken with a little bit of water, moving it often so it doesn't stick.
6. Place sliced chicken on a plate with cucumber-tomato salad.

Zucchini Pasta

PREP TIME	COOK TIME	CALORIES
15 Min	10 Min	245

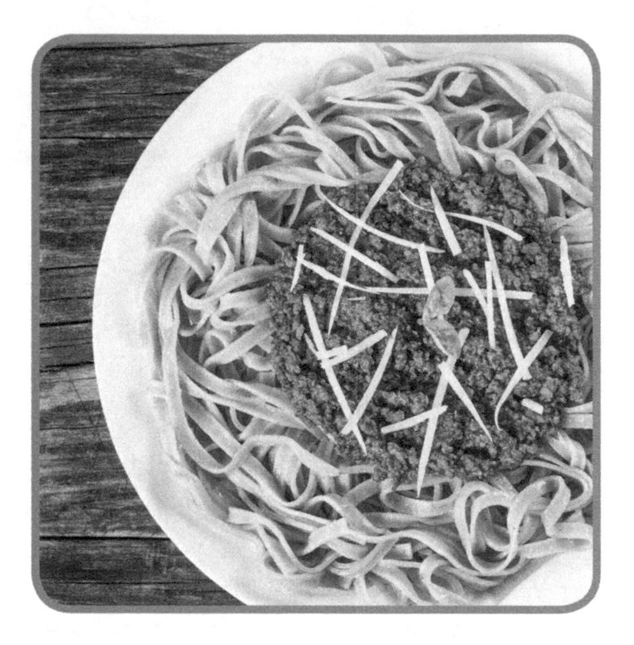

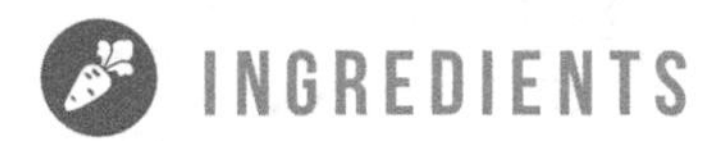

INGREDIENTS

100g lean ground beef (95% lean)

1 large zucchini

1 cup tomatoes, chopped

1 garlic clove, finely minced

Fresh basil

Sea salt & pepper to taste

DIRECTIONS

1. Place a box grater on its side with the largest grating holes facing up.
2. Cut the ends of the zucchini, and then push along the top of the grater in long strokes to create long, thin ribbons of zucchini.
3. In a large non-stick pan, add minced garlic, chopped tomato, basil and salt & pepper.
4. Add ground beef and break apart with a cooking spoon. Cook until no longer pink.
5. Add zucchini and cook until slightly tender.
6. Serve with fresh basil on top.

Shrimp on Cauliflower Rice

PREP TIME	COOK TIME	CALORIES
15 Min	**15 Min**	**245**

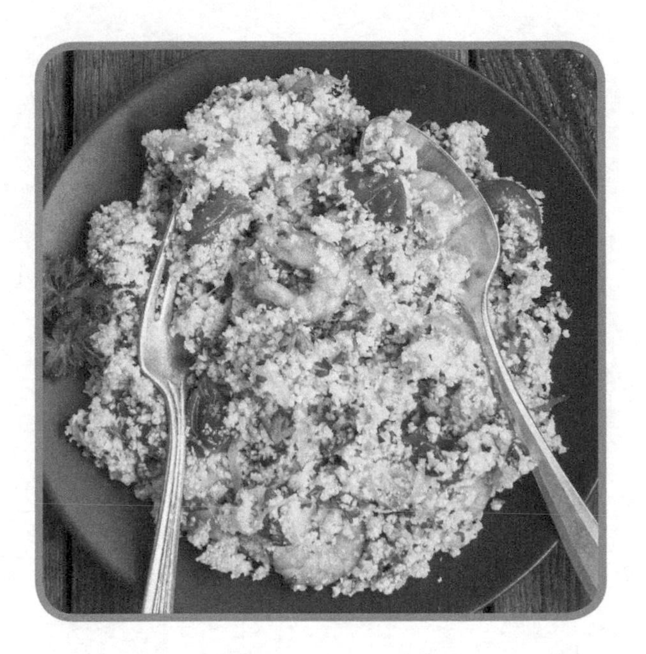

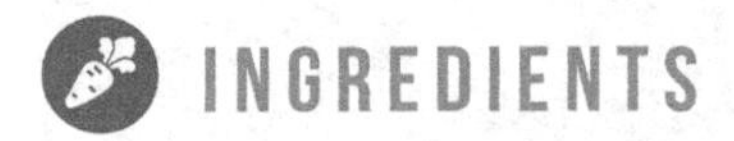

INGREDIENTS

150g uncooked shrimp

1 small cauliflower

1 cup broccoli

1 garlic clove, finely minced

4 tbsp. soy sauce

1 tsp. garlic power

DIRECTIONS

1. Wash and cut the cauliflower into large pieces.
2. Transfer the cauliflower to a food processor and pulse until completely broken down. It should be processed until it looks like pieces of rice.
3. In a non-stick frying pan over medium heat, add water, processed cauliflower, chopped broccoli, garlic, and soy sauce. Mix thoroughly and cook for 3-5 minutes.
4. Place in a separate non-stick frying pan over medium heat.
5. Cook the shrimp with a little bit of water until nicely pink and cooked. Season with salt and garlic powder.
6. Serve cauliflower on a plate with shrimp on top.

Pork Chops & Bok Choy

PREP TIME	COOK TIME	CALORIES
5 Min	**15 Min**	**263**

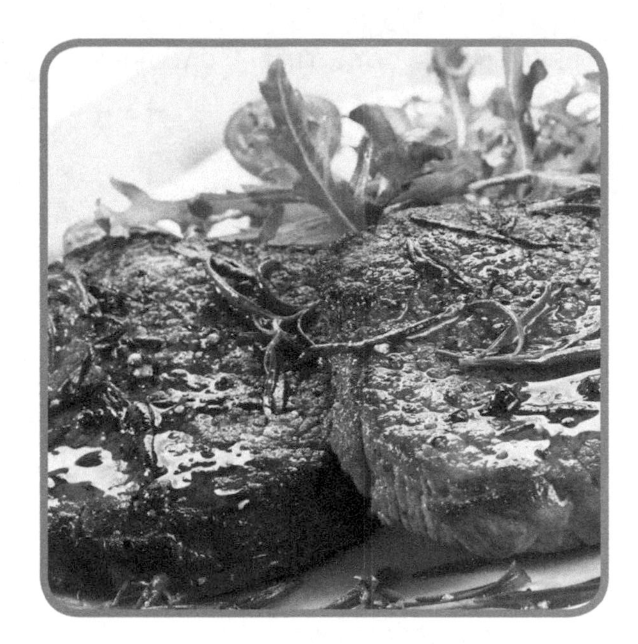

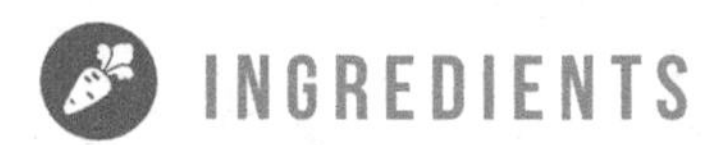

INGREDIENTS

1 pork chop

3 cups of bok choy

1 garlic clove, finely minced

Sea salt & pepper to taste

DIRECTIONS

1. Season pork chop with salt and pepper.
2. Place in a non-stick frying pan over medium heat. Move the pan around quickly so it doesn't stick. Add water as needed. Wait until seared and flip.
3. Once pork chop is cooked, remove from pan. Don't discard the oil left in pan.
4. Add chopped bok choy and garlic to pan. Cook until tender. Add salt to taste.
5. Add pork chop back to pan with bok choy to re-heat and absorb juices.

Turkey Taco Lettuce Wraps

PREP TIME	COOK TIME	CALORIES
5 Min	10 Min	252

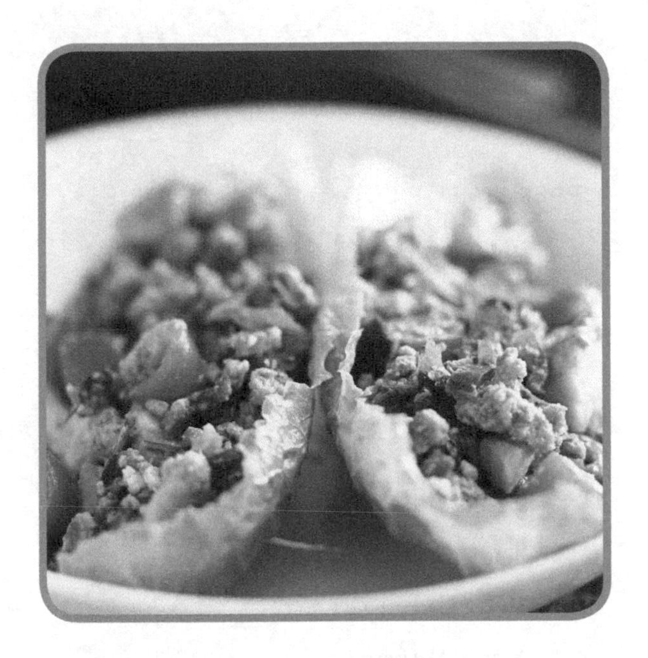

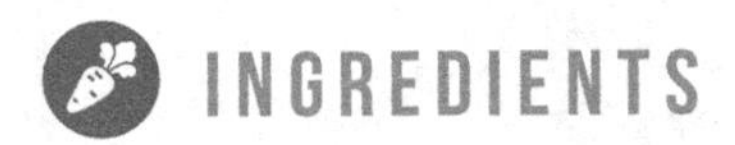

INGREDIENTS

150g extra-lean ground turkey breast

1 tsp. garlic powder

1 tsp. cumin

1 tsp. salt

1 tsp. chili powder

1 tsp. paprika

½ tsp. oregano

½ small onion, minced

8 large iceberg lettuce leaves

DIRECTIONS

1. Brown turkey in large non-stick skillet over medium heat, breaking into smaller pieces as it cooks.
2. When no longer pink, add dry seasonings and mix well.
3. Add the onion, pepper, water, and cover. Simmer on low for about 20 minutes.
4. Wash and dry the lettuce. Divide meat equally between the eight leaves and place in the center of each leaf.
5. Wrap each leave and pin with toothpick to hold in place.

FastTrack Dinners

Fish & Zucchini Chips

PREP TIME	COOK TIME	CALORIES
5 Min	20 Min	243

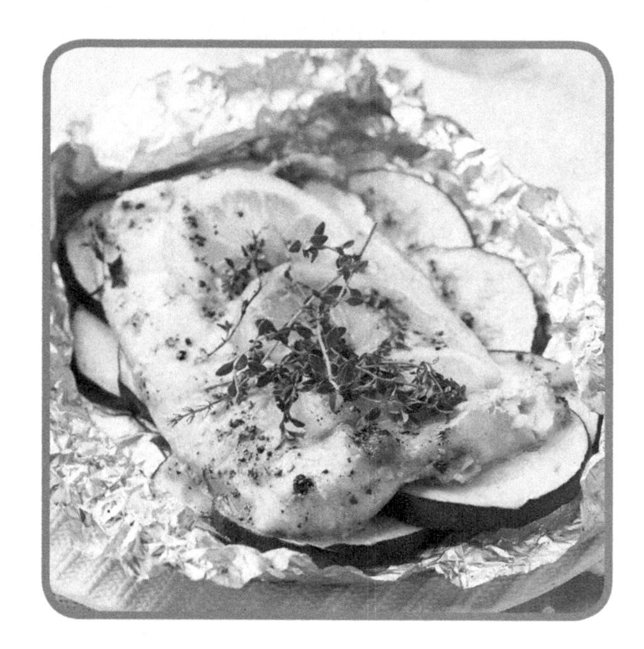

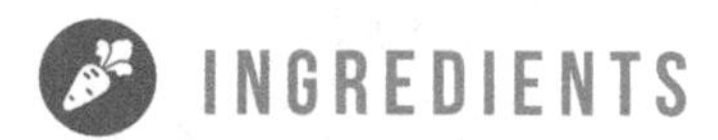

INGREDIENTS

1 cod fillet (approximately 220g)

1 large zucchini

½ fresh lemon

1 tsp. thyme

Sea salt & pepper to taste

DIRECTIONS

1. Preheat oven to 400°F.
2. Cut off the ends of the zucchini and slice remaining portion into thin pieces like chips – the thinner the better.
3. Place wax paper in non-stick, Pyrex glass cooking sheet.
4. Lay zucchini flat, spread out evenly, and season with salt and pepper to taste. Bake for 15 minutes.
5. In a separate cooking sheet, place cod in the center and season with salt and pepper to taste.
6. Squeeze lemon over the cod, sprinkle thyme, and bake for 10 minutes.
7. Remove cod and zucchini when browned and serve.

Beef Stir-Fry on Cauliflower Rice

PREP TIME	COOK TIME	CALORIES
10 Min	**15 Min**	**274**

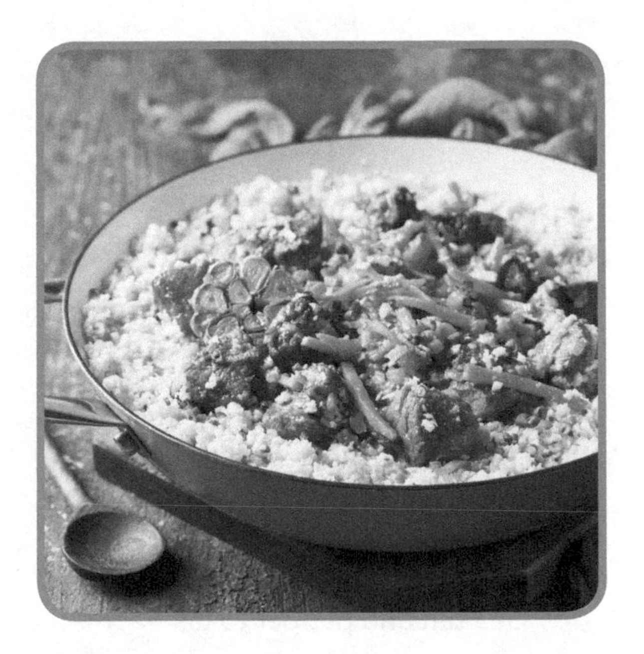

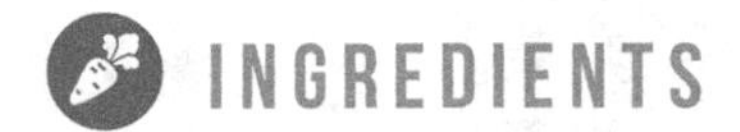

INGREDIENTS

100g flank steak

1 small cauliflower

½ cup green onion

1 garlic clove, finely minced

4 tbsp. soy sauce

DIRECTIONS

1. Season strip steak with salt and pepper.
2. Place steak on non-stick frying pan over medium heat, moving the pan around quickly so it doesn't stick. Wait until seared and flip.
3. Once done, remove steak and cut into thin slices. Add chopped onions and garlic and cook until soft.
4. While that's cooking, wash and cut the cauliflower into large pieces.
5. Transfer the cauliflower to a food processor and pulse until completely broken down. It should be processed until it looks like pieces of rice.
6. Add processed cauliflower to same frying pan as steak to keep the juices. Add chopped steak and soy sauce. Mix thoroughly and cook for 3-5 minutes.
7. Serve cauliflower on a plate with steak on top.

Lettuce Burger

PREP TIME	COOK TIME	CALORIES
10 Min	**20 Min**	**256**

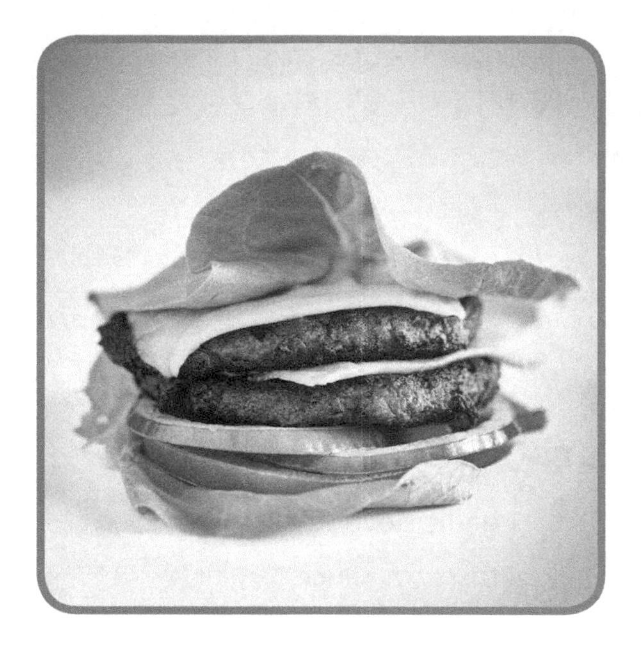

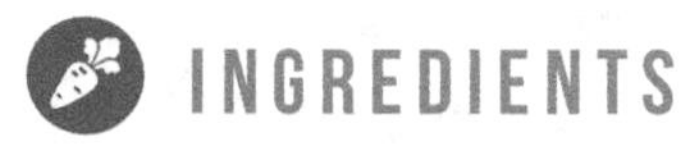

INGREDIENTS

150g extra lean ground beef (95% lean)

1 head of lettuce

1 tomato

1 red onion

Sea salt and pepper to taste

DIRECTIONS

1. Preheat oven to 400°F.
2. In a medium bowl, mix ground beef, ½ a diced onion, and salt & pepper to taste.
3. Roll mixture into patties and place in non-stick Pyrex glass cooking sheet.
4. Bake for 10 minutes per side.
5. Cut lettuce into three parts, keeping the outside halves for the buns. Slice remaining onion and tomato.
6. Assemble burger and enjoy.

Chicken Breast & Cucumber

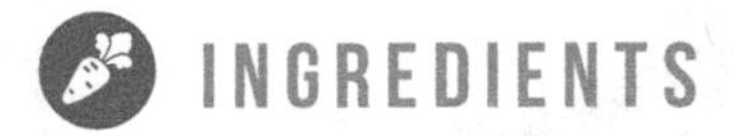

PREP TIME	COOK TIME	CALORIES
5 Min	**20 Min**	**261**

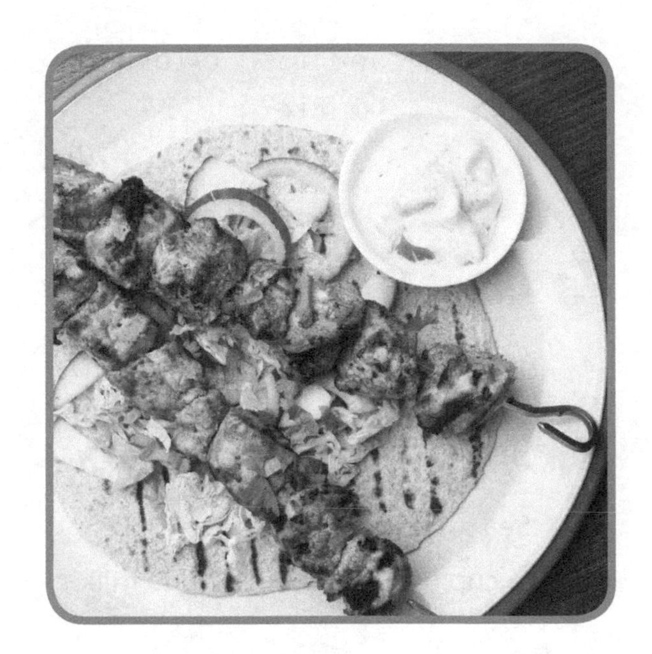

INGREDIENTS

130g extra lean chicken breast

1 large cucumber

3 tsp. vinegar

Sea salt & pepper to taste

DIRECTIONS

1. Cut chicken into three strips and place skewers through each.
2. Season chicken with salt and pepper.
3. Place chicken on BBQ and cook thoroughly. Tip: Rub the side of a cut onion on the grill to prevent sticking.
4. Chop cucumber into slices and mix with vinegar. Salt and pepper to taste.
5. Serve chicken over cucumber salad.

Lamb Chops & Brussels

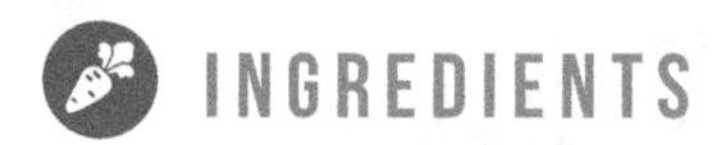

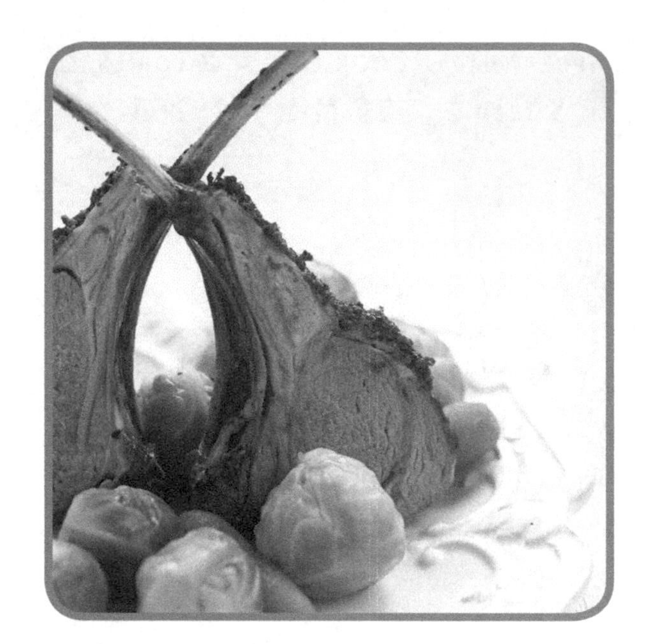

INGREDIENTS

100g leg of lamb (fat trimmed off)

1 cup brussel sprouts

½ red pepper

Sea salt & pepper to taste

¼ cup unsweetened almond milk

DIRECTIONS

1. Season lamb with salt and pepper.
2. Place lamb on non-stick frying pan over medium heat, moving the pan around quickly so it doesn't stick.
3. Once cooked, add brussel sprouts and sliced red pepper. Cook until tender.
4. Season with sea salt and pepper to taste and serve.

Turkey & Mashed Cauliflower

PREP TIME	COOK TIME	CALORIES
10 Min	**20 Min**	**253**

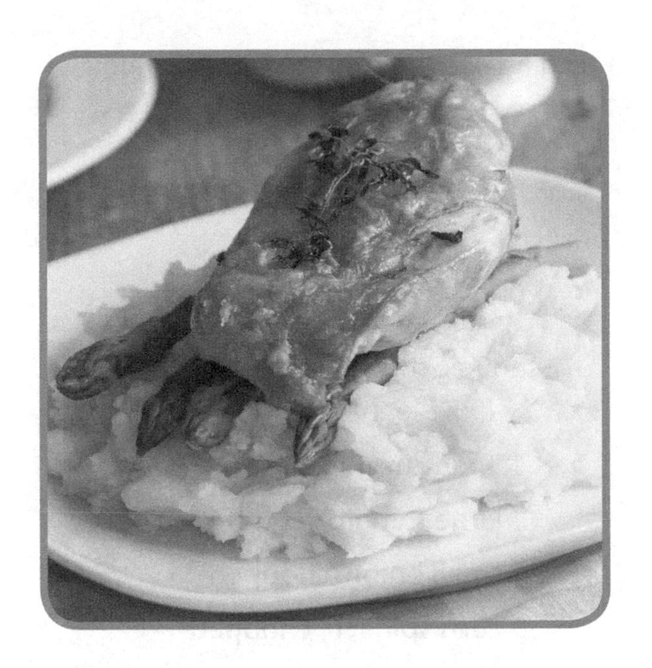

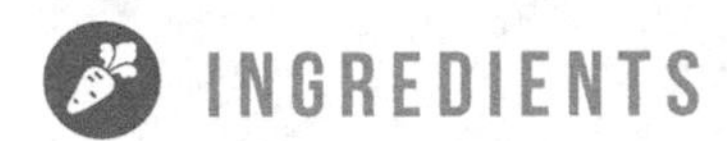

INGREDIENTS

100g extra lean turkey breast

1 small whole cauliflower

2 cups asparagus

2 tbsp. chives

Sea salt and pepper to taste

DIRECTIONS

1. Season turkey with salt and pepper.
2. Place turkey on non-stick frying pan over medium heat, moving the pan around quickly so it doesn't stick.
3. Once cooked, add asparagus with trimmed ends. Season to taste and cook until tender.
4. In another pot, boil cauliflower until very tender.
5. Drain and discard all the water – the drier the cauliflower the better.
6. Add almond milk, salt and pepper, and mash with potato masher until it looks like mashed potatoes.
7. Top with chives.

Zucchini Lasagna

PREP TIME	COOK TIME	CALORIES
10 Min	**1 Hour**	**277**

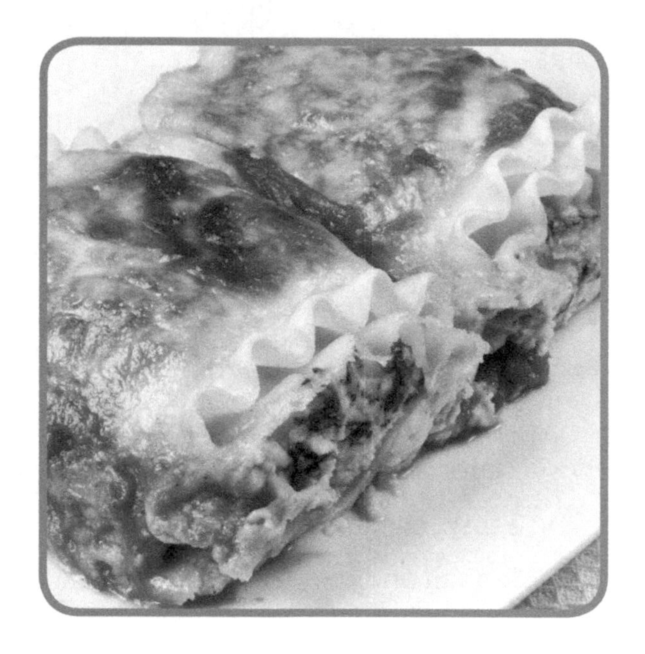

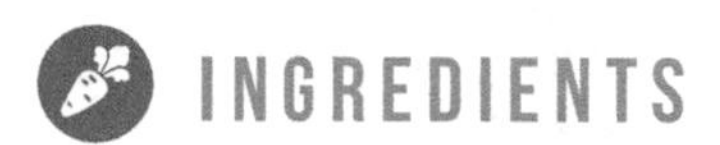

INGREDIENTS

- 100g extra lean ground beef (95% lean)
- 1 large zucchini
- 1 large tomato
- 1 small onion, chopped
- 3 cups spinach, chopped
- 2 tbsp. fresh basil
- 1 tbsp. fresh oregano
- 1 tbsp. salt
- 1 tbsp. pepper

DIRECTIONS

1. Preheat oven to 325°F.
2. Slice zucchini lengthwise into very thin slices. Cut tomato into thin slices.
3. In a large non-stick skillet over medium-high heat, mix ground beef, chopped onion, spinach, spices, and water and cook for 15 minutes.
4. To assemble lasagna, spread ⅓ of the meat sauce in the bottom of a Pyrex glass cooking sheet. Then layer ⅓ the zucchini slices, and ⅓ of the tomato slices. Repeat layering until you have used all the ingredients.
5. Bake for 45 minutes covered with foil. Let stand 5 minutes before serving.

FastTrack Soups

Vegan "Chicken" Noodle Soup

PREP TIME	COOK TIME	CALORIES
10 Min	0	75

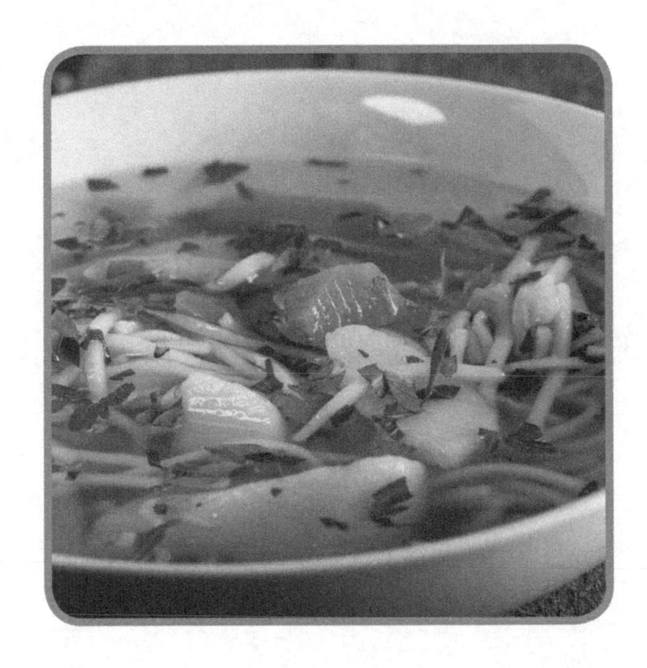

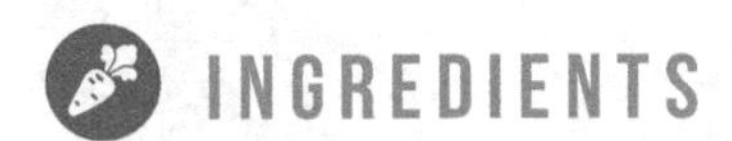

INGREDIENTS

2 cups of water

1 cup cauliflower, chopped

1 cup celery

1 small zucchini, shaved

2 cloves of garlic, minced

2 tbsp. fresh parsley

Sea salt & pepper to taste

DIRECTIONS

1. Add to blender – water, cauliflower, celery, parsley, garlic, and salt. Blend and add more water if necessary. You can warm the soup with the heat of your blender.
2. Place a box grater on its side with the largest grating holes facing up.
3. Cut the ends of the zucchini, and then push along the top of the grater in long strokes to create long, thin ribbons of zucchini.
4. Add zucchini ribbons to warm soup and serve.

All-Vegetable Soup

PREP TIME	COOK TIME	CALORIES
10 Min	**0**	**68**

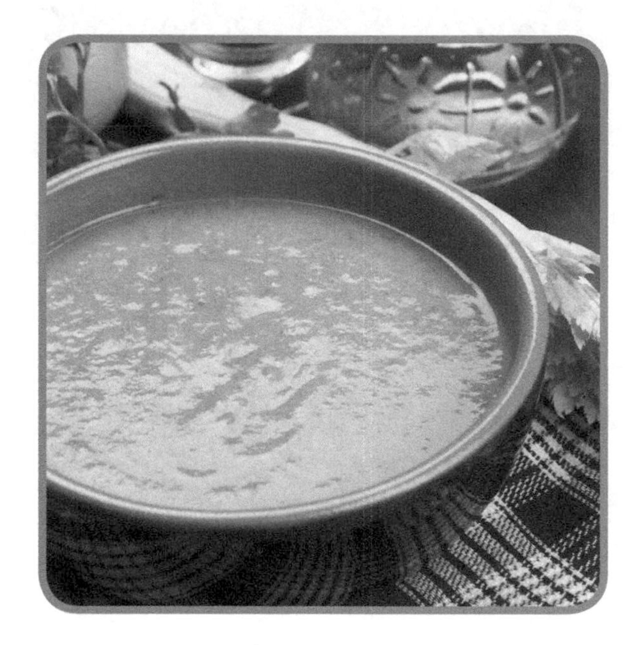

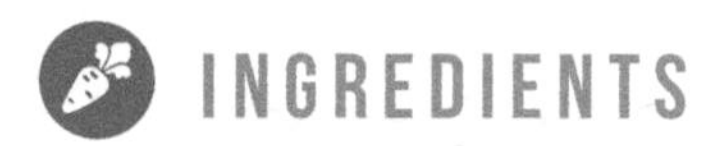

INGREDIENTS

2 cups water

1 cup chopped broccoli

2 cups chopped cauliflower

1 cup celery

1 cup spinach

2 cloves of garlic, minced

Sea salt & pepper to taste

DIRECTIONS

1. Add to blender – water, broccoli, cauliflower, celery, spinach, garlic, and salt & pepper. Blend and add more water if necessary. You can warm the soup with the heat of your blender.

Homemade Tomato Soup

PREP TIME	COOK TIME	CALORIES
10 Min	**0**	**60**

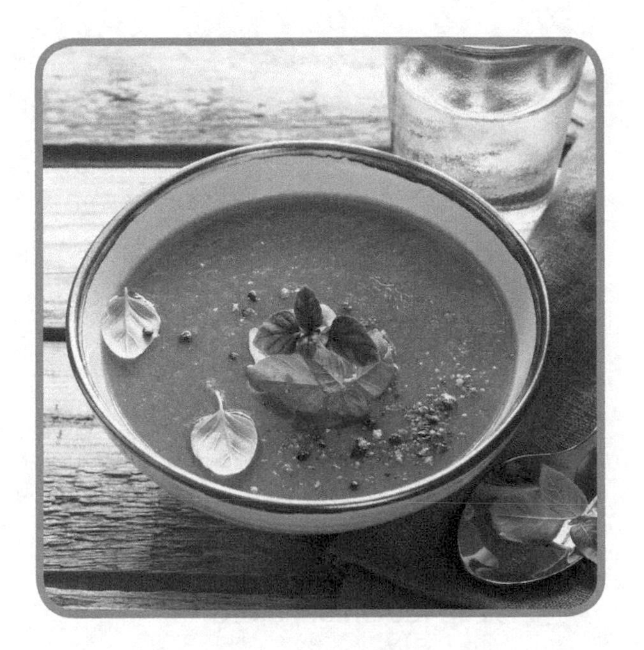

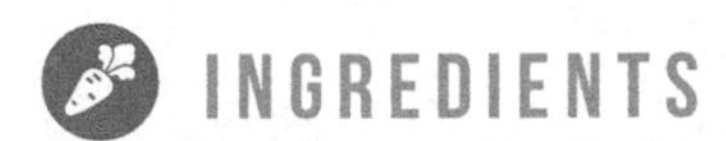

INGREDIENTS

1 small onion, chopped

1 cup tomatoes, chopped

2 cloves of garlic, minced

2 tsp. unsweetened balsamic vinegar

½ tsp. dried thyme

Sea salt & pepper to taste

DIRECTIONS

1. Add to blender – onion, tomatoes, garlic, vinegar, thyme, and salt & pepper. Blend and add more water if necessary. You can warm the soup with the heat of your blender.

Slow & Steady

Simple Spring Salad

PREP TIME	COOK TIME	SERVES
10 Min	0	2

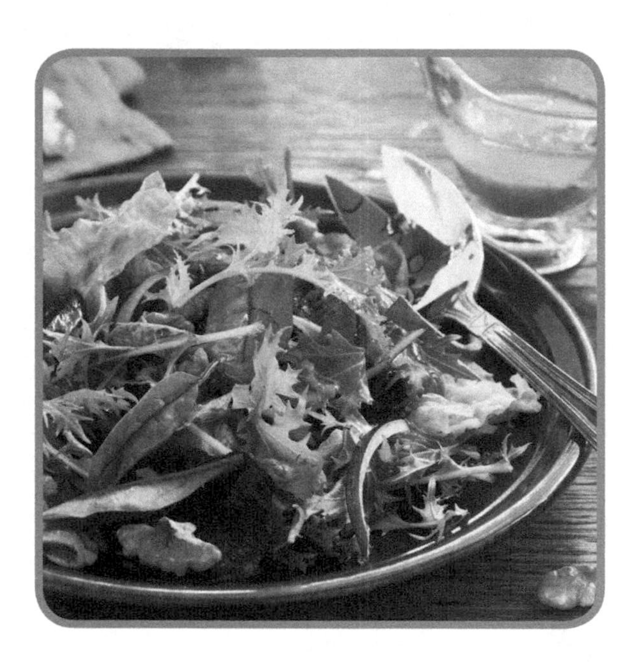

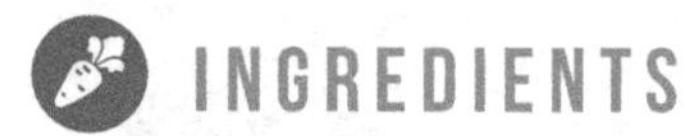

INGREDIENTS

1 cup extra virgin olive oil

1 bag of spring salad mix

¼ cup red onion, diced

2 cloves garlic, minced

2 oz. roasted pecans

1 tbsp. Dijon mustard

3 tbsp. balsamic vinegar

½ tsp. black pepper

½ tsp. sea salt

DIRECTIONS

1. Blend all ingredients except olive oil and pecans in a high-speed blender or food processor until smooth.
2. Once smooth, slowly add in the olive oil to fully emulsify.
3. Serve atop your choice of salad.
4. Sprinkle with roasted pecans and serve.

Simple Coleslaw

PREP TIME	COOK TIME	SERVES
10 Min	**0**	**2**

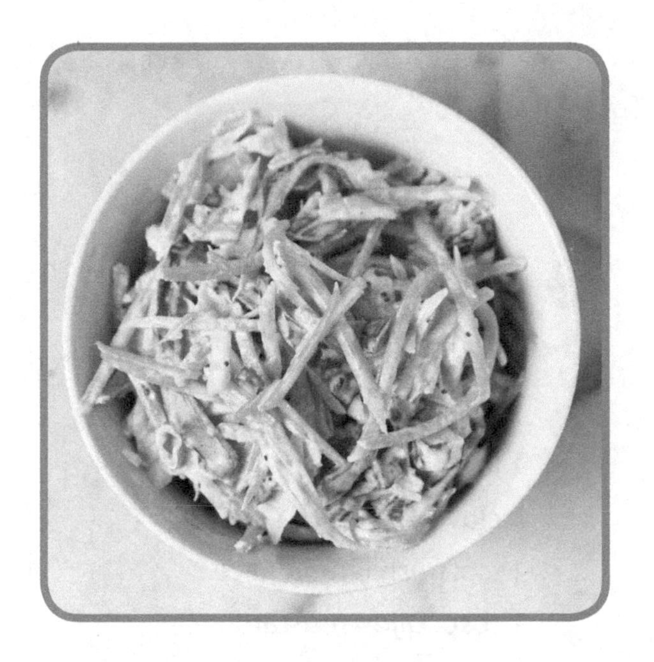

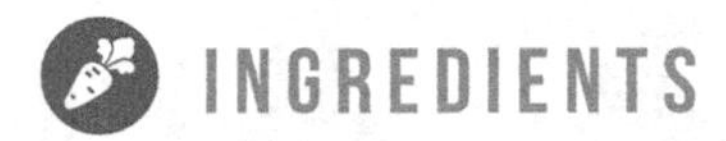

INGREDIENTS

1 cup extra virgin olive oil

1 bag of coleslaw salad mix

¼ cup red onion, diced

2 cloves garlic, minced

2 oz. roasted pecans

1 tbsp. Dijon mustard

3 tbsp. balsamic vinegar

½ tsp. black pepper

½ tsp. sea salt

DIRECTIONS

1. Blend all ingredients except olive oil and pecans in a high-speed blender or food processor until smooth.
2. Once smooth, slowly add in the olive oil to fully emulsify.
3. Serve atop your choice of salad.
4. Sprinkle with roasted pecans and serve.

Creamy Caesar Salad

PREP TIME	COOK TIME	SERVES
10 Min	0	2

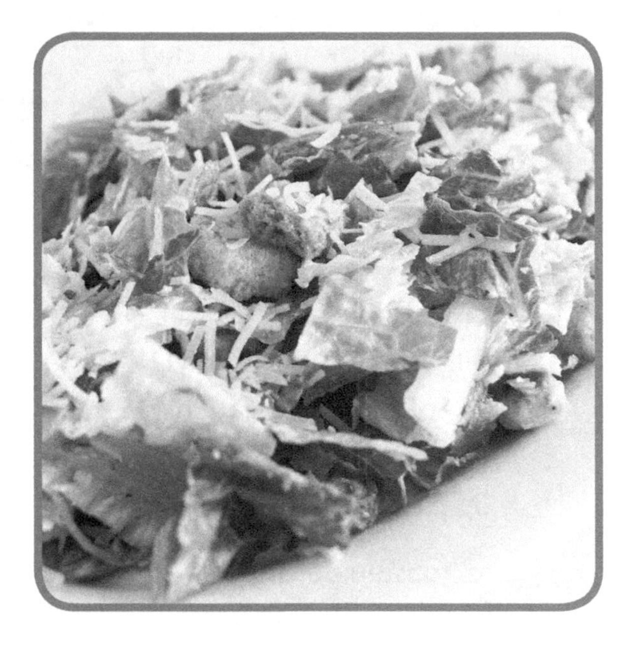

INGREDIENTS

3 hearts of romaine lettuce, chopped

1 ripe avocado, diced

1 large egg

3 cloves garlic, smashed

1 tsp. fresh lemon juice

1 tbsp. Dijon mustard

⅓ cup of avocado oil

2 tbsp. raw cashew pieces

Sea salt & black pepper to taste

DIRECTIONS

1. Add egg, two garlic cloves, lemon juice, mustard, oil, and salt and pepper to a tall glass jar that's barely wide enough to accommodate the head of your immersion blender and let it sit until the egg settles at the bottom.
2. Insert your immersion blender and push it all the way down until it touches the bottom of the jar.
3. Push the power button and do not move the blender. This will cause dressing to emulsify and become thick and creamy. Blend for approximately 20 seconds.
4. Add cashews, remaining garlic clove, and salt to a food processor and give them a few quick pulses until texture resembles that of grated parmesan.
5. Add lettuce, avocado, and dressing to a large mixing bowl.
6. Toss to combine.
7. Divide salad between four plates and sprinkle with parmesan-like mixture.
8. Serve immediately.

Creamy Dill Cucumber Salad

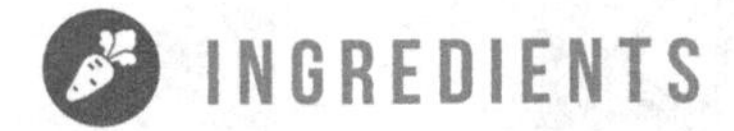

PREP TIME	COOK TIME	SERVES
10 Min	0	1

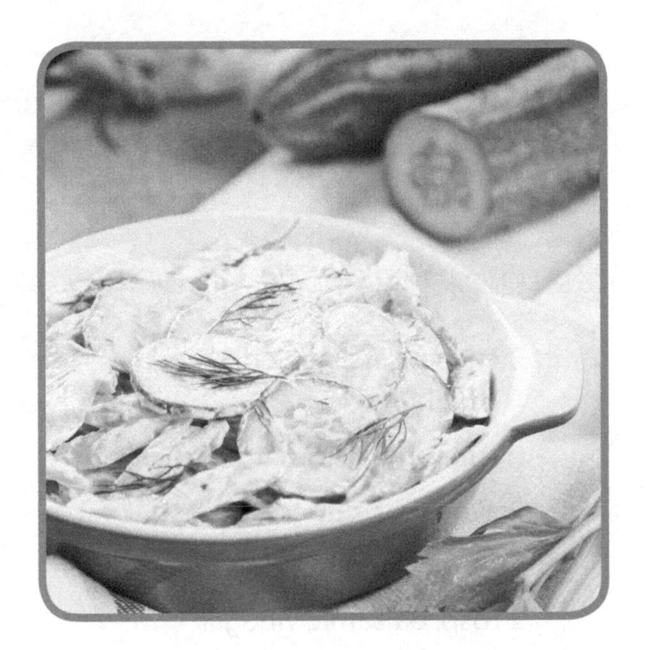

INGREDIENTS

4 mini cucumbers

¼ cup of mayonnaise

2 tbsp. fresh dill, finely chopped

1 tbsp. extra virgin olive oil

½ tsp. Dijon mustard

Sea salt & pepper to taste

DIRECTIONS

1. In a small bowl, combine all the ingredients, except for the cumbers, and mix well with a fork.
2. Pour over the sliced cucumbers and stir delicately until well combined.
3. Optional: Cover and place in fridge for two hours to allow flavors to meld.

Tomato, Cucumber, Avocado Salad

PREP TIME	COOK TIME	SERVES
10 Min	0	1

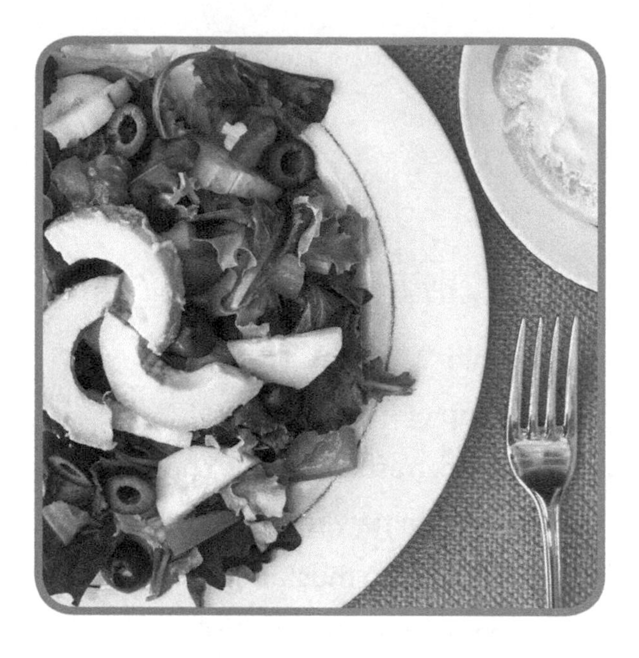

INGREDIENTS

3 cucumbers, peeled, sliced, and halved

2 cups cherry tomatoes, sliced

2 avocados, cubed

¼ cup olive oil

2 tbsp. balsamic vinegar

1 tbsp. dried oregano

2 tsp. dried basil leaf

Sea salt & pepper, to taste

DIRECTIONS

1. Wash veggies. Peel and slice cucumber and tomatoes.
2. Place in a large bowl and sprinkle with parmesan cheese (optional).
3. In a separate small bowl, add olive oil, balsamic vinegar, oregano, basil, salt and pepper. Mix well.
4. Pour dressing over veggies and mix.
5. Place in refrigerator until ready to serve.
6. Add avocados just before serving.
7. Enjoy!

Crunchy Kale Salad

PREP TIME	COOK TIME	SERVES
15 Min	**0**	**1**

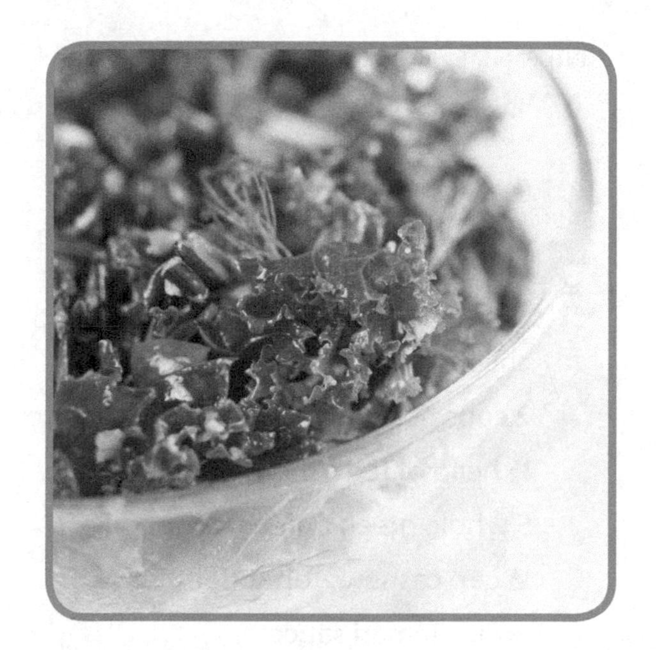

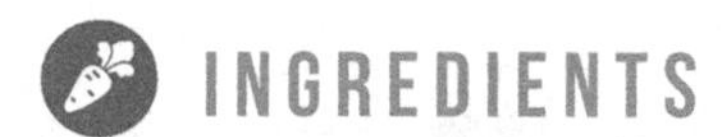

INGREDIENTS

1 bunch kale

½ cup red cabbage, shredded

1 lemon, juiced

Zest of 1 lemon

1 tbsp. olive oil

¼ cup nuts, chopped

Sea salt & pepper to taste.

DIRECTIONS

1. Cut the kale leaves thinly down the middle along the vein, stack, and thinly slice into ribbons. Place in a large bowl.
2. Add the shredded red cabbage, lemon juice and zest, olive oil, salt, and pepper to the kale. Stir thoroughly to combine.
3. For best results, allow the salad to sit for at least 30 minutes before serving. The veggies will soften just a bit.
4. Top with chopped nuts for a bit more crunch.

Asian Salad

PREP TIME	COOK TIME	SERVES
10 Min	0	2

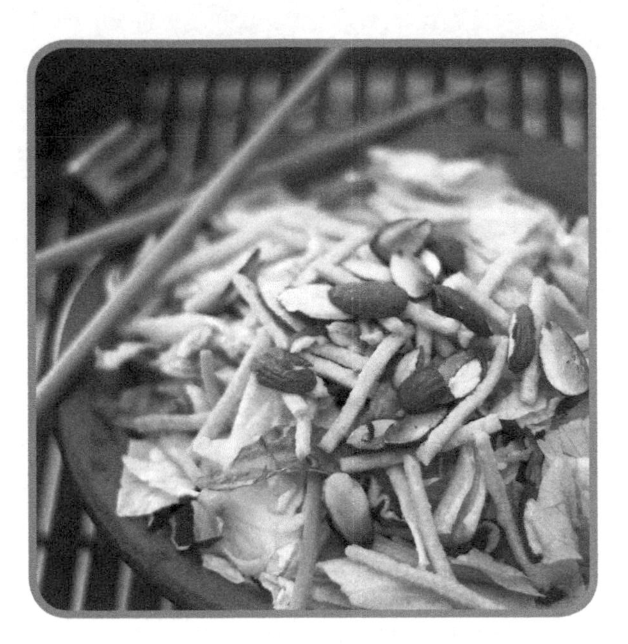

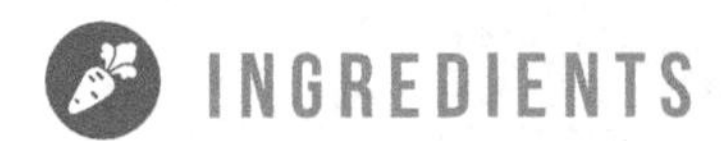

INGREDIENTS

chicken, torn into shreds

2 cups head lettuce, shredded

½ head of red cabbage, shredded

5 whole green onions, chopped

½ cup cashews (optional)

¼ cup Tamari sauce

¼ cure white wine vinegar

2 tbsp. finely minced ginger

3 tbsp. extra virgin olive oil

2 tbsp. Hoisin sauce

1 tbsp. whhite sesame seeds, 1 tbsp. black sesame seeds

Sea salt & pepper to taste

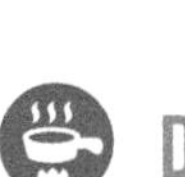

DIRECTIONS

1. In a small mason jar with lid, add tamari, vinegar, minced ginger, olive oil, hoisin sauce, sea salt, and chopped green onions. Secure the lid and shake vigorously. Set aside.
2. Next, put chopped lettuce, cabbage, sesame seeds, cashews, and enough dressing to coat (around half) into a large plastic bag. Seal and shake vigorously until well incorporated. Adjust amount of dressing as needed.
3. Place on a plate and top with remaining dressing.

Meatloaf

PREP TIME	COOK TIME	SERVES
10 Min	**25 Min**	**4**

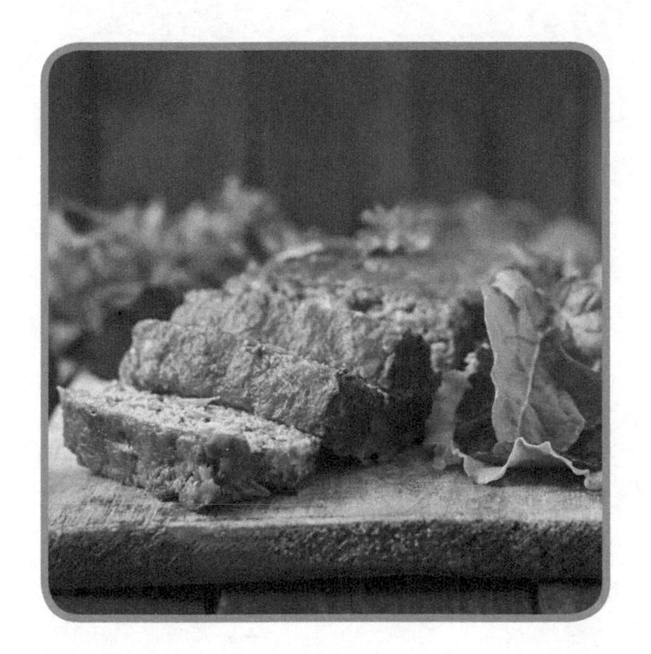

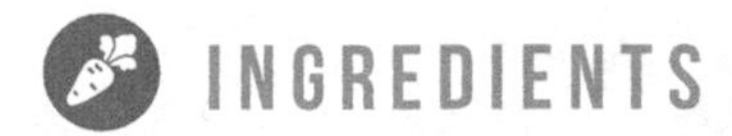

INGREDIENTS

1 lb. ground beef

½ onion, finely chopped

½ green pepper, finely chopped

1 tbsp. chili powder

2 tbsp. Worcestershire sauce

2 egg whites

2 tbsp. Dijon mustard

DIRECTIONS

1. Preheat oven to 400°F. Crumble ground beef into a large bowl.
2. Add chopped onion, green pepper, Worcestershire sauce, and Dijon mustard. Stir with fork.
3. Add eggs and stir again until well blended. You may need to use your hands.
4. Spoon mixture into prepared muffin pan. Bake for 25 minutes.

Pesto Chicken & Tomato Kebabs

PREP TIME	COOK TIME	SERVES
40 Min	**10 Min**	**6**

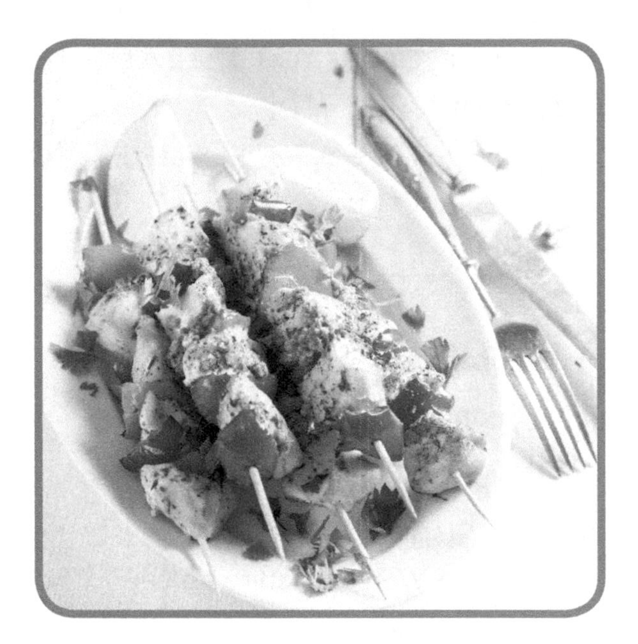

INGREDIENTS

2 lbs. chicken, cut into 1-inch cubes

24 cherry tomatoes

1 clove of garlic

1 cup fresh basil leaves, chopped

Sea salt & pepper to taste

DIRECTIONS

1. In a food processor, pulse basil, garlic, salt, and pepper until smooth.
2. In a bowl, combine the raw chicken with pesto and marinate for a few hours. Soak wooden skewers in water at least 30 minutes (or use metal ones to avoid this step). Beginning and ending with chicken, thread chicken and tomatoes onto eight pairs of parallel skewers to make eight kebabs total.
3. Heat the outdoor grill or indoor grill pan over medium heat until hot. Be sure the grates are clean. Place kebabs on the hot grill and cook about 3-4 minutes; turn and continue cooking until chicken is cooked throughout, about 2-3 minutes.
4. Serve and enjoy!

Garlic-Lime Pork Chops

PREP TIME	COOK TIME	SERVES
25 Min	**10 Min**	**4**

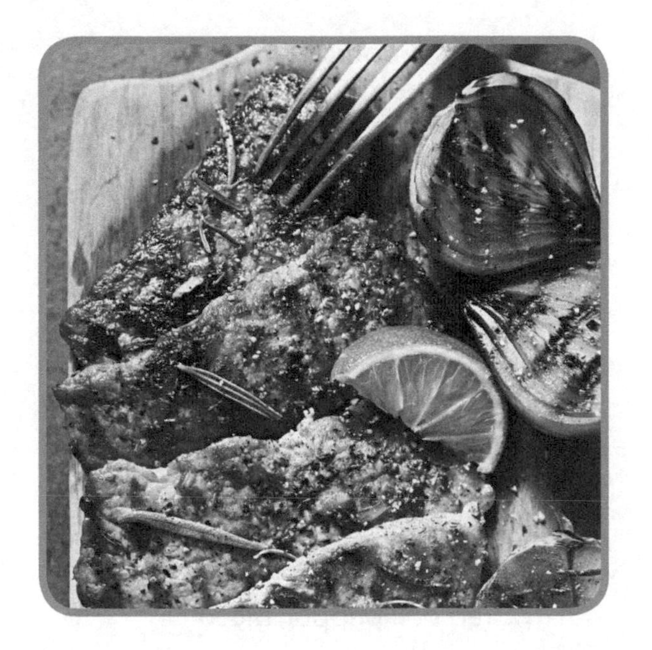

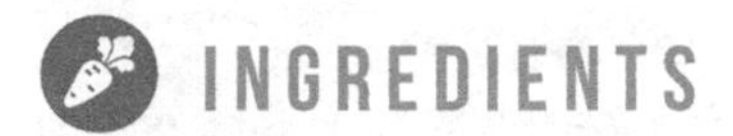

INGREDIENTS

4 pork chops

4 cloves garlic, crushed

1 tsp. cumin

1 tsp. chili powder

1 tsp. paprika

Sea salt & pepper to taste

½ lime, juiced

DIRECTIONS

1. In a large bowl, season pork with garlic, cumin, chili powder, paprika, salt, and pepper. Squeeze lime juice over the meat, add some zest from the lime, and let it marinade at least 20 minutes.
2. Line broiler pan with foil for easy clean up. Place pork chops on the broiler pan and broil about 4-5 minutes on each side or until nicely browned.

Summer Veggies & Sausage

PREP TIME	COOK TIME	SERVES
10 Min	20 Min	4

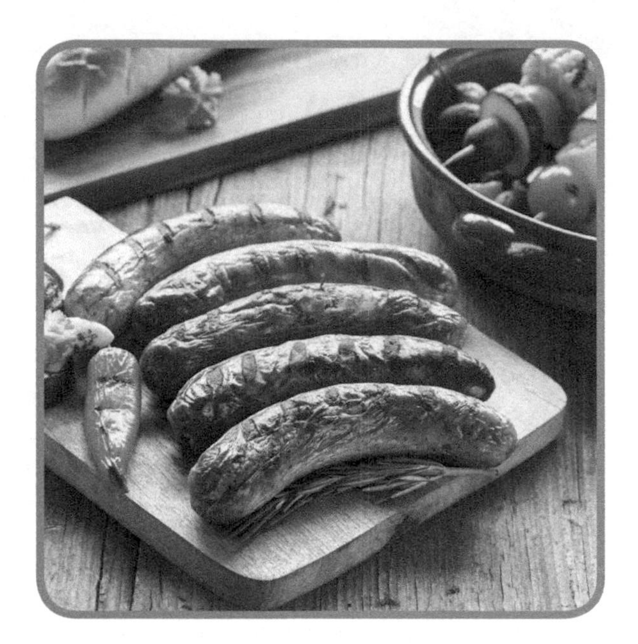

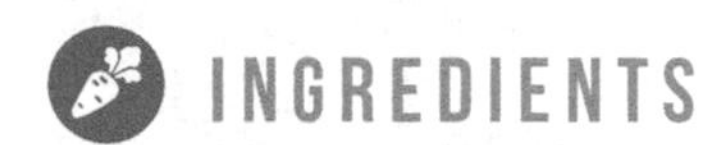

INGREDIENTS

14 oz. Italian sausage, sliced 1-inch thick

1 large onion, chopped

½ orange bell pepper, diced

½ yellow bell pepper, diced

½ red bell pepper, diced

2 cups zucchini, ½-inch thick & quartered

4 cloves garlic, smashed

2 tbsp. fresh rosemary

Sea salt & pepper to taste.

DIRECTIONS

1. Add sausage to the skillet and sauté over medium-low heat, stirring occasionally until browned but not quite cooked through, about 10 minutes.
2. Season chopped vegetables with salt and pepper. Add onions, peppers, garlic, and rosemary to the skillet and mix.
3. Continue cooking, stirring occasionally until onions and peppers become slightly browned.
4. Add zucchini and cook an additional 5 minutes, mixing as it cooks until cooked throughout.

Bacon & Eggs

PREP TIME	COOK TIME	SERVES
0	**10 Min**	**1**

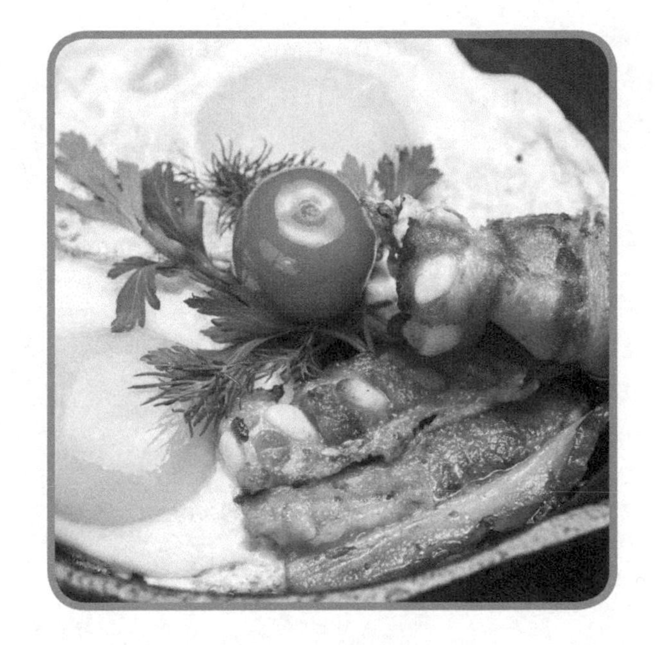

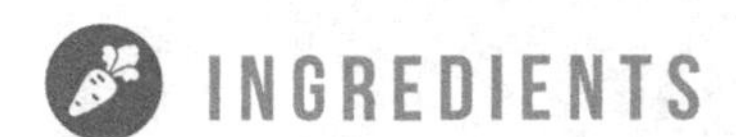

INGREDIENTS

3 eggs

4 slices bacon, cooked

Sea salt & pepper to taste

DIRECTIONS

1. Using a large skillet, place slices of bacon in pan over medium-high heat. Turn down the heat as soon as the bacon starts to sizzle.
2. Cook it while turning every couple of minutes until it reaches the crispness you desire.
3. Drain bacon on a plate layered with paper towels.
4. Once it's cooked, turn down the heat to medium-low. Don't drain the bacon fat – use it to fry your eggs.
5. Crack three eggs into the pan. Use a slotted spatula to remove the eggs from the pan.
6. Blot each egg with paper towel before putting it on a plate with bacon.
7. Salt & pepper to taste.

Grilled Rosemary Lamb Chops

PREP TIME	COOK TIME	SERVES
1 Hour	20 Min	4

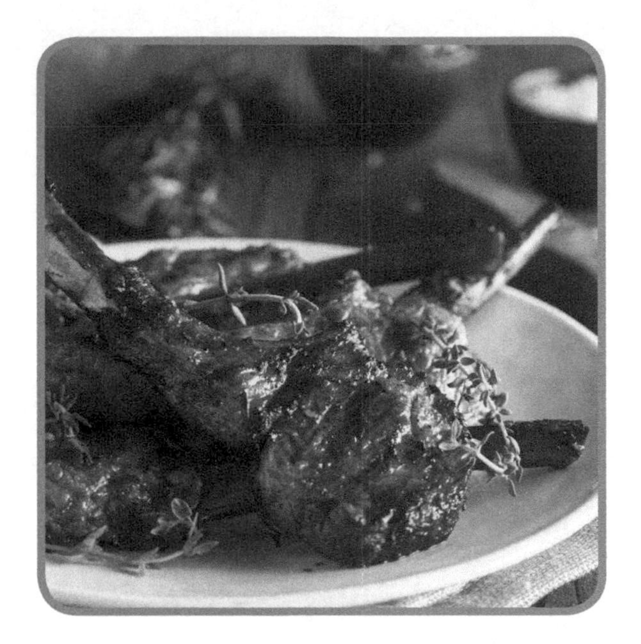

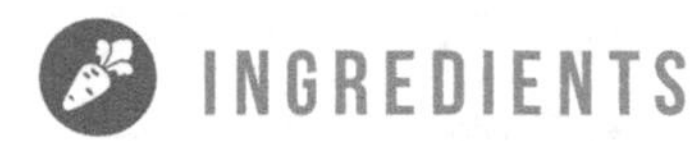

INGREDIENTS

4 lamb chops

3 cloves of garlic

¼ cup fresh lemon juice

1 tbsp. fresh rosemary leaves

Sea salt & pepper to taste

DIRECTIONS

1. Combine lemon juice, garlic, and rosemary.
2. Season lamb with salt & pepper and cover with garlic mixture.
3. Marinate at least one hour, overnight if possible.
4. Discard marinade and grill over medium-high heat to desired liking or broil in the oven.

BBQ Ribs

PREP TIME	COOK TIME	SERVES
5 Min	90 Min	4

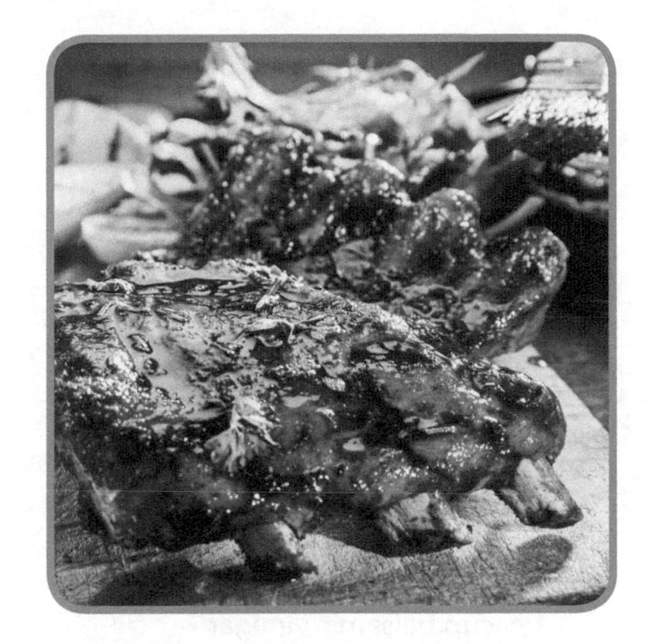

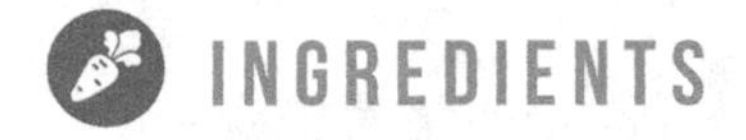

INGREDIENTS

4 lbs. baby back pork ribs

Cayenne pepper

Garlic powder

Sea salt & pepper to taste

DIRECTIONS

1. Preheat grill on high heat.
2. Place ribs on large sheet of heavy-duty aluminum foil.
3. Mix all the spices together to make a dry rub.
4. Rub all sides of the ribs with spice mixture.
5. Place ribs in foil on the grill and cook for one hour.
6. Remove ribs from foil and place directly on grill for 30 additional minutes.

Balsamic Roast Beef

PREP TIME	COOK TIME	SERVES
30 Min	6 Hours	8

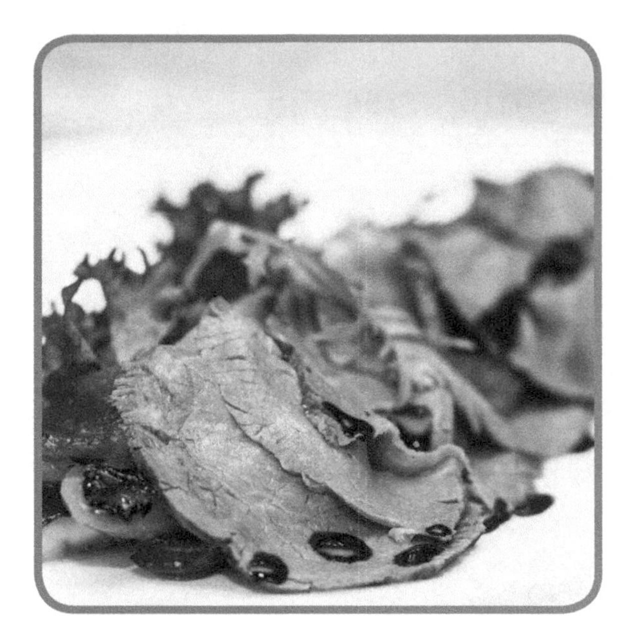

INGREDIENTS

3 lbs. boneless beef chuck roast

1 onion, sliced

2 sprigs of fresh rosemary

2 bay leaves

2 cloves of garlic, minced

⅓ cup balsamic vinegar

1 ½ cups beef stock

Sea salt & black pepper to taste

DIRECTIONS

1. Season the roast on all sides with sea salt & black pepper.
2. Melt some cooking fat in a large skillet over medium-high heat and sear the roast for 2-3 minutes on each side.
3. Place the meat in a slow cooker and top with onion, garlic, balsamic vinegar, beef stock, bay leaves, and rosemary. Cover the slow cooker, turn on low, and cook for six hours.
4. Remove and discard the two bay leaves and rosemary sprigs.
5. Pour the liquid from the slow cooker into a saucepan and bring to a slow boil over medium-high heat until you get the desired consistency for your sauce.
6. Pour the sauce back in the slow cooker and serve with the meat and vegetables.

Butterflied, Roasted Chicken

PREP TIME	COOK TIME	SERVES
15 Min	**1 Hour**	**4**

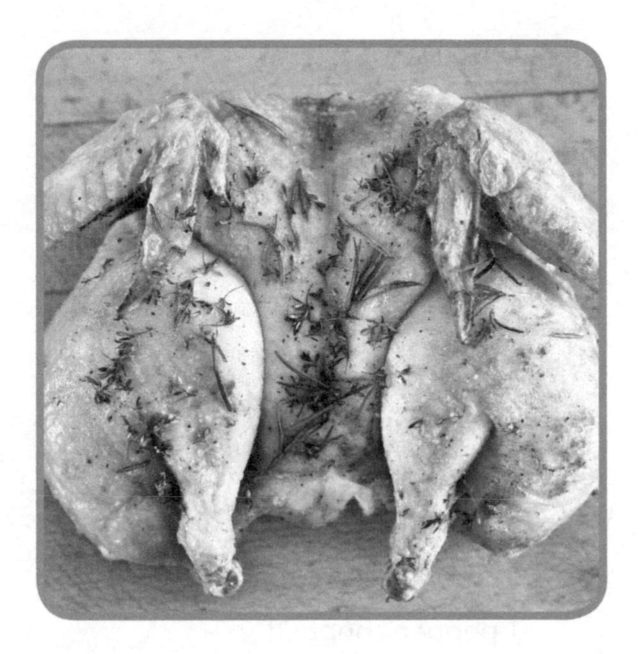

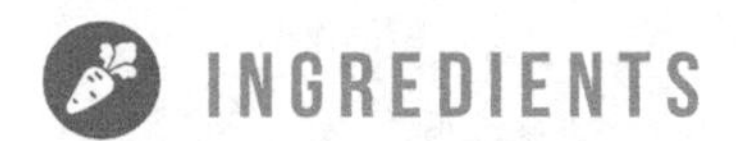

INGREDIENTS

1 whole chicken

2 onions, peeled and quartered

1 zucchini, sliced

2 bell peppers, chopped

2 lemons, halved

3 tbsp. fresh rosemary, finely chopped

Sea salt & pepper to taste

DIRECTIONS

1. Preheat oven to 400°F.
2. Place the chicken breast-side down on cutting board. Cut along both sides of the backbone from end to end with kitchen shears and remove the backbone. Flip the chicken and open it like a book. Press firmly on the breasts with your palm to flatten.
3. Place the chicken in Pyrex baking sheet and surround with vegetables and lemon.
4. Season chicken and vegetables with rosemary, salt, and pepper to taste.
5. Place baking sheet in the oven and cook for an hour.

Bean-Less Chili

PREP TIME	COOK TIME	SERVES
10 Min	**30 Min**	**8**

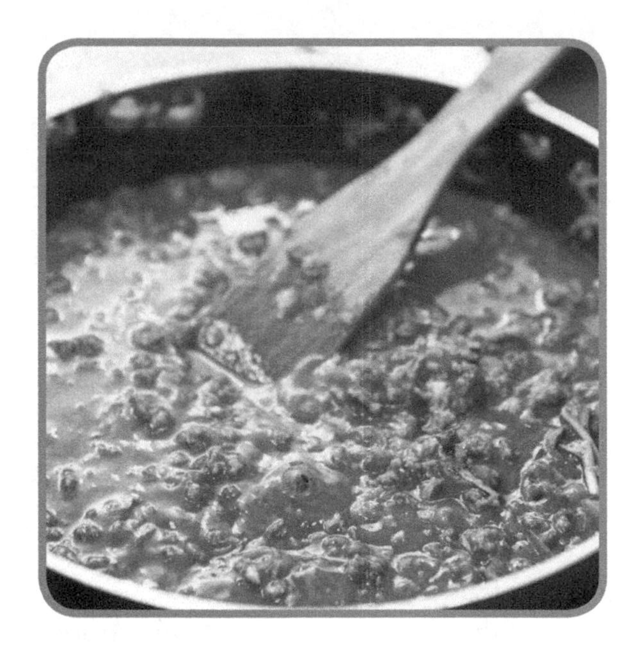

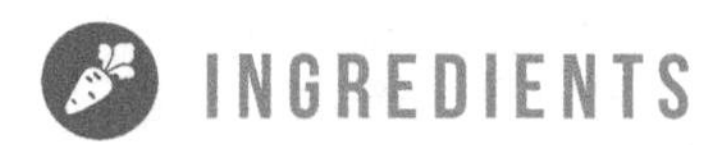

INGREDIENTS

5 lbs. ground beef

2 cups water

1 cup tomatoes

1 onion, finely chopped

5 celery stalks, chopped

1 pepper, chopped

4 cups button mushrooms, chopped

1 tbsp. extra-virgin olive oil

4 bay leaves, 3 thyme sprigs, 2 tbsp. fresh parsley

Sea salt & pepper to taste

DIRECTIONS

1. In a large skillet over a medium heat, cook the ground beef with some cooking fat if needed.
2. In a very large saucepan over a medium heat, sauté the garlic in olive oil. Cook for about two minutes or until the garlic is fragrant.
3. Add the onion, celery, pepper, tomatoes, and mushrooms to the saucepan. Stir well and cook for another 5-10 minutes until vegetables are soft.
4. Add the cooked ground beef and bay leaves, thyme, and parsley. Stir well.
5. Season to taste with salt and pepper, reduce heat to low, and simmer uncovered for about four hours or until thick, stirring occasionally.
6. Adjust the seasoning by adding salt or pepper if needed, and remove the bay leaves and thyme sprigs.

Quick Fish Curry

PREP TIME	COOK TIME	SERVES
10 Min	**20 Min**	**4**

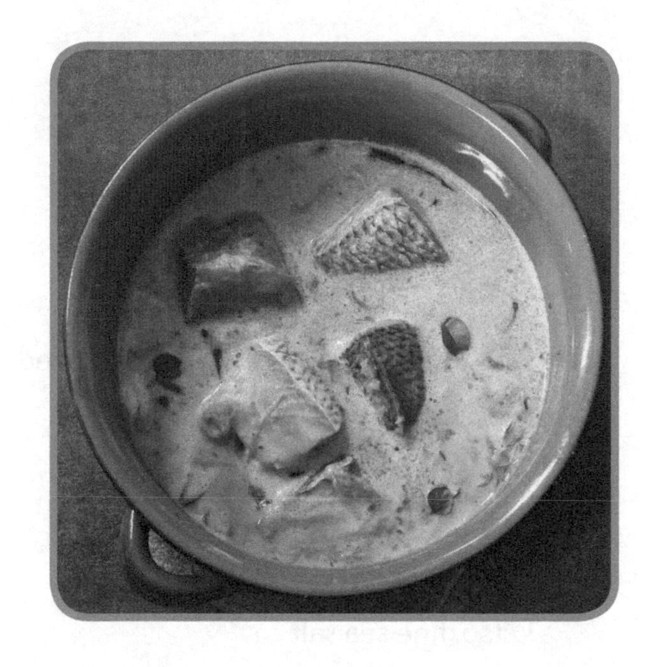

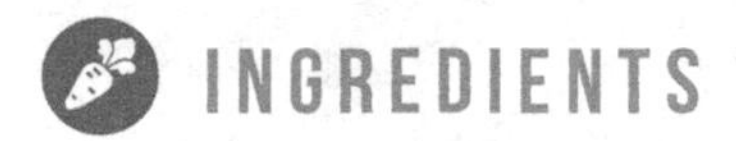

INGREDIENTS

20 oz. fish, cut into 1-inch chunks

1 onion, finely chopped

2 tomatoes, chopped

3 cloves garlic, thinly sliced

2 tbsp. freshly grated ginger

2 tbsp. coconut oil

2 tsp. medium curry powder

1 tsp. ground turmeric

10 leaves of curry and coriander

12 oz. coconut milk

Sea salt

DIRECTIONS

1. Melt the coconut oil in a medium saucepan.
2. Sauté the onion over a medium heat until translucent and just starting to brown.
3. Add the garlic and ginger and cook for one minute.
4. Add the turmeric, curry powder, and curry leaves.
5. Continue to cook for one minute, and then slowly stir in the coconut milk. Bring to a simmer.
6. Add the chopped tomatoes and simmer for five minutes until the tomatoes begin to soften.
7. Add the fish, season to taste with salt, and gently poach for 6-8 minutes until the fish is cooked. Gently stir in the coriander and lime juice.
8. Serve with cauliflower rice.

Baked Avocado Fries

PREP TIME	COOK TIME	SERVES
10 Min	15 Min	2

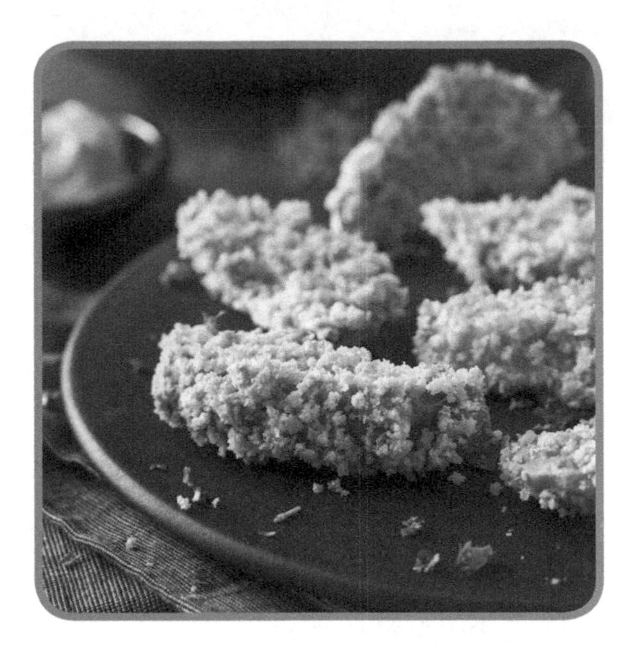

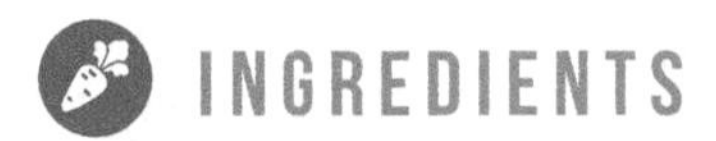

INGREDIENTS

2 ripe but firm avocados, pits removed

1 large egg, beaten

2 tsp. garlic powder

1 tsp. onion powder

1 tsp. paprika

½ tsp. fine sea salt

½ tsp. black pepper

⅓ cup arrowroot (tapioca) flour

1 tsp. stone ground mustard

1-½ cups crushed pork rinds

DIRECTIONS

1. Preheat the oven to 425°F (218°C) and line a baking sheet with foil.
2. Slice the avocados in half and carefully remove the pit. Cut each half into three or four slices and set them aside.
3. You'll need three small bowls for the dipping stations. In the first bowl, combine the arrowroot and half the seasonings. In the second, combine the beaten egg, water, and mustard. In the third, combine the pork rinds and the other half of the seasonings.
4. Dip the avocado slices in the arrowroot, then the eggs, and then the pork rinds. Lay them on the baking sheet. When they're all dipped, bake the avocado fries for 10-12 minutes, then flip, and bake another 2-4 minutes. They're best enjoyed while they're fresh!

Spicy Chicken Bites

PREP TIME	COOK TIME	SERVES
20 Min	40 Min	4

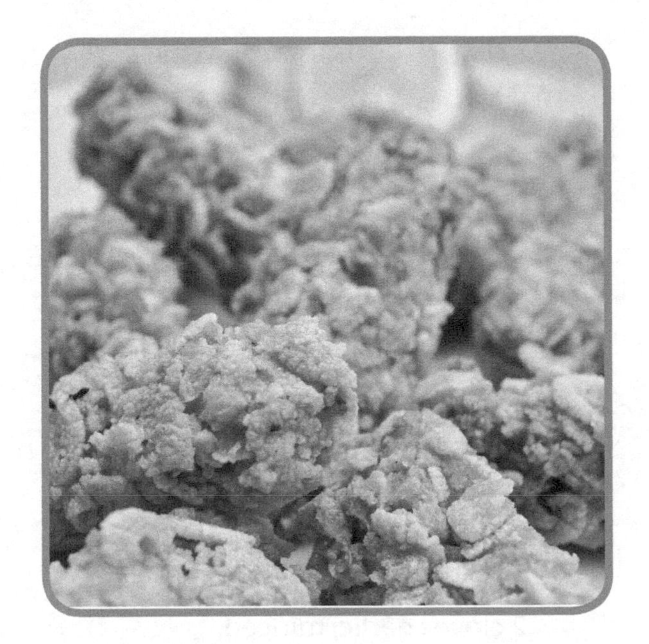

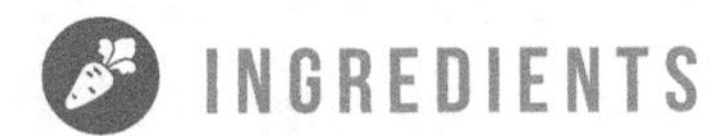

INGREDIENTS

1 lbs. chicken tenders

2 eggs

2 ¼ cups almond flour

¼ cup tapioca or potato starch

½ tsp. sea salt

¼ tsp. fresh cracked pepper

½ tsp. garlic powder

⅓ cup unsweetened hot sauce

(Franks brand works great!)

DIRECTIONS

1. Preheat the oven to 425°F. Line a rimmed baking sheet with parchment paper.
2. Place the almond flour, garlic powder, sea salt, and fresh cracked pepper in a bowl and mix together. Place the eggs in another bowl with a splash of water and whisk them.
3. Dip the chicken tenders, one at a time, into the tapioca or potato starch, then into the egg, and then into the almond flour. Lay the chicken tenders on the prepared baking sheet. Bake the chicken for 40 minutes or until crispy and beginning to get golden brown.
4. Serve with hot sauce as a dipping sauce.

Shepherd's Pie

PREP TIME	COOK TIME	SERVES
30 Min	**30 Min**	**6**

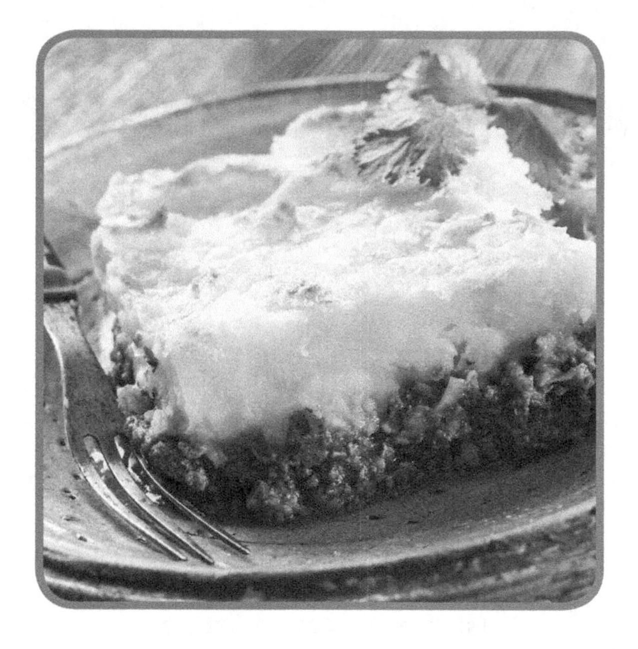

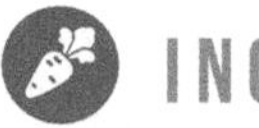

INGREDIENTS

1 lbs. ground beef

1 small onion, diced

2 celery ribs, diced

1 pepper, diced

1 head of cauliflower, chopped

2 cloves garlic, minced

½ cup beef broth

2 tbsp. parsley, chopped

Sea salt & pepper to taste

DIRECTIONS

1. Preheat the oven to 400°F. Grease a 2-3 quart casserole dish and set aside.
2. In a large pot, steam or boil cauliflower until tender.
3. In a large skillet or saucepan over medium high heat, add the onion, celery, pepper, and garlic and cook until beginning to soften, around five minutes.
4. Add the ground meat to the pan and cook until browned. Add beef broth as necessary to keep the mixture wet. Add the ketchup or tomato paste (if using), parsley, and season with salt and pepper. Let simmer while you prepare the cauliflower topping.
5. To make the topping, drain the cooked cauliflower. Mash or puree with a stick blender until smooth. Add two tablespoons of fat; season with salt and pepper.
6. To assemble, spread the meat mixture on the bottom of the dish. Top with the cauliflower mixture and smooth with a spoon. Cover with shredded cheese, if desired.
7. Bake for 30 minutes or until the top is brown and bubbly. Serve warm.

CITATIONS

1. Global Report On Diabetes. *WHO.* [Online] 2016.
http://www.who.int/diabetes/global-report/en/.

2. Diabetes Atlas Sixth Edition. *IDF.* [Online] 2014.
http://www.idf.org/diabetesatlas/update-2014.

3. National Diabetes Statistics Report. *CDC.* [Online] 2014.
http://www.cdc.gov/media/releases/2014/p0610-diabetes-report.html.

4. Diabetes Treatments: World Drug Market 2013-2023. [Online] Visiongain, 2013.
http://www.visiongain.com/Report/1033/Diabetes-Treatments-World-Drug-Market-2013-2023.

5. New Analysis Concludes Cause of Diabetes Not Genetic. *Diabetes In Control.* 2010.
http://www.diabetesincontrol.com/new-analysis-concludes-cause-of-diabetes-not-genetic/.

6. Glucose Control And Vascular Complications In Veterans With Type 2 Diabetes. *New England Journal Of Medicine.* [Online] 2009.
http://www.nejm.org/doi/full/10.1056/NEJMoa0808431#t=article.

7. Antidepressants: Benefits of Reboxetine Not Proven. *Institute For Quality & Efficiency In Health Care.* [Online] 2009.
https://www.iqwig.de/en/press/press-releases/press-releases/antidepressants-benefit-of-reboxetine-not-proven.2405.html.

8. UK Prospective Diabetes Study. *University Of Oxford.* [Online] 1999.
https://www.dtu.ox.ac.uk/UKPDS/trialresults.php.

9. List Of Largest Pharmaceutical Settlements. *Wikipedia.* [Online]
https://en.wikipedia.org/wiki/List_of_largest_pharmaceutical_settlements.

10. Insulin: Undertanding Its Action In Health And Disease. *Oxford Journal.* [Online] 2000.
http://bja.oxfordjournals.org/content/85/1/69.full.pdf+html.

11. Myth: Insulin Is Needed For Glucose Uptake. *Nadeem J Qureshi.* [Online] 2012.
http://nadeem.no/2012/10/07/glucose-uptake-is-not-insulin-dependant/.

REFERENCES

1. **Very Low Calorie Diet in Type 2 Diabetes (Newcastle University)**
Taylor R MD (2014) Type 2 diabetes mellitus is generally regarded as an irreversible chronic condition. As a very low calorie diet can bring about…
http://www.ncl.ac.uk/magres/research/diabetes/documents/VerylowcaloriedietS.Stevenetal.pdf

2. **Pathogenesis of Type 2 Diabetes: Tracing the Reverse Route… (PubMed)**
Taylor R MD (2008) The metabolic abnormalities of type 2 diabetes can be reversed reproducibly by bariatric surgery. By quantifying the major…
https://www.ncbi.nlm.nih.gov/pubmed/18726585

3. **Reversal of Type 2 Diabetes: Normalisation of Beta Cell Function… (PubMed)**
Taylor R MD (2011) Type 2 diabetes is regarded as inevitably progressive, with irreversible beta cell failure. The hypothesis was tested that both beta cell…
https://www.ncbi.nlm.nih.gov/pubmed/21656330

4. **Population Response To Information On Reversibility… (Newcastle University)**
Taylor R MD (2013) Following publication of the Couterpoint Study on the reversibility of Type 2 diabetes using a very low energy diet, the extent of public…
http://www.ncl.ac.uk/magres/research/diabetes/documents/CounterpointReflections.pdf

5. **Reversing The Twin Cycles Of Type 2 Diabetes… (Newcastle University)**
Taylor R MD (2012) It has become widely accepted that Type 2 diabetes is inevitably life-long, with irreversible and progressive beta cell damage…
http://www.ncl.ac.uk/magres/research/diabetes/documents/BantingDiabeticMed.pdf

6. **Insulin Independent Glucose Transport Regulates Insulin Sensitivit… (PubMed)**
Ebeling P (1998) The glucose transport proteins (GLUT1 and GLUT4) facilitate glucose transport into insulin-sensitive cells. GLUT1 is insulin independent…
https://www.ncbi.nlm.nih.gov/pubmed/9801136

7. **Functional Properties And Genomics Of Glucose Transporter (PubMed)**
Zhao FQ (2007) Glucose is the major energy source for mammalian cells as well as an important substrate for protein and lipid synthesis. Mammalian cells…
https://www.ncbi.nlm.nih.gov/pubmed/18660845

8. **A Comparison Of Basel And insulin Stimulated Glucose Transport… (PubMed)**
Ludvigsen C (1980) Specific D-glucose transport in plasma membranes prepared from control and insulin treated rat adipocytes was measure using a recently…
https://www.ncbi.nlm.nih.gov/pubmed/6991329

9. **Estimation And Kinetic Analysis Of insulin Independent Glucose... (PubMed)**
Gottesman I (1983) Using the glucose clamp technique, glucose uptake was determined isotopically in normal human volunteers at plasma glucose...
https://www.ncbi.nlm.nih.gov/pubmed/6344653

10. **An Analysis Of How To Measure Glucose During Glucose Clamps... (PubMed)**
Hompesch M (2008) This article provides a perspective on the challenges of appropriate glucose measurement in the context of glucose clamp experiments.
https://www.ncbi.nlm.nih.gov/pubmed/19885275

11. **The Contribution Of Insulin Dependent And Insulin Independent... (PubMed)**
Kahn SE (1994) Glucose disposal occurs by both insulin independent and insulin dependent mechanisms, the latter being determined by the interaction of...
https://www.ncbi.nlm.nih.gov/pubmed/8138065

12. **Fasting Hyperglycemia In Non-insulin-Dependent Diabetes Mellitu... (PubMed)**
DeFronzo RA (1989) The factors responsible for fasting hyperglycemia were investigated in 77 normal weight non-insulin-dependent diabetic and 72 Age...
https://www.ncbi.nlm.nih.gov/pubmed/2657323

13. **Hyperglycemia-Induced Stimulation Of Glucose Transport In Skele... (PubMed)**
Huang HM (2012) A physiologically based model proposed by our group has been developed to assess glucose transport and phosphorylation in skeletal...
https://www.ncbi.nlm.nih.gov/pubmed/22986442

14. **Cardiac And Adipose Tissue Abnormalities But Not Diabetes In... (PubMed)**
Katz (1985) The insulin-sensitive glucose transporter, GLUT4, is the most abundant facilitative glucose transport in muscle and adipose tissue, the...
https://www.ncbi.nlm.nih.gov/pubmed/7675081

15. **Normal Muscle Glucose Uptake In Mice Deficient In Muscle GLUT4 (PubMed)**
Fam BC (2012) Skeletal muscle insulin resistance is a major characteristic underpinning type 2 diabetes. Impairments in the insulin responsiveness...
https://www.ncbi.nlm.nih.gov/pubmed/22736482

16. **insulin, Growth Hormone And Sport (PubMed)**
Sonksen PH (2001) This review examines some interesting 'new' histories of insulin and reviews our current understanding of its physiological actions ...
https://www.ncbi.nlm.nih.gov/pubmed/11431133

17. **Biological Active Ingredients Of Traditional Chinese Herb Astragalu... (PubMed)**
Zhang K (2015) Diabetes mellitus is a serious chronic metabolic disease which disease afflicting at present no afflicts approximately 4% of world population...
https://www.ncbi.nlm.nih.gov/pubmed/25723453

18. **Effects Of Astragalus Membranaceus Extract On Diabetic Nephrapa... (PubMed)**
Kim J (2014) Diabetic nephropathy, a microvascular complication of diabetes, is a progressive kidney disease caused by angiopathy of the capillaries in the kidney...
https://www.ncbi.nlm.nih.gov/pubmed/25298884

19. **Characterization And Hypoglycemic Effect Of A Polysaccharide ... (PubMed)**
Zhu J (2013) Diabetes mellitus is a group of complicated metabolic disorders characterized by high blood glucose level and inappropriate insulin secreting...
https://www.ncbi.nlm.nih.gov/pubmed/23987311

20. **The Protective Effects Of Lycium Barbarum And Chrysanthemum... (PubMed)**
Hu CK (2012) the effects of Lycium barbarum and Chrysanthemum morifolum extracts on diabetic retinopathy were evaluated. The diabetes model was...
https://www.ncbi.nlm.nih.gov/pubmed/22487267

21. **Hypoglycemic And Hypolipidemic Effects And Antioxidand Activity... (PubMed)**
Luo Q (2004) The hypoglycemic and hypolipidemic effects of Lycium babarum fruit water decoction, crude polysaccharide extracts, and purified polysaccharide...
https://www.ncbi.nlm.nih.gov/pubmed/15519360

22. **The Effects of Enriched Chicory Inulin on Liver Enzymes, Calcium... (PubMed)**
Farhangi MA (2016) Type 2 diabetes mellitus as one of the main causes of morbidity and mortality is associated with immune system disturbances...
https://www.ncbi.nlm.nih.gov/pubmed/26872721

23. **Effects of the Extracts from Roasted Chicory (Cichorium Intybus L)... (PubMed)**
Nishimur M (2015) The extract from roasted chicory root, which contains inulin-type fructans, has favorable effects including anti-hyperglycemic and...
https://www.ncbi.nlm.nih.gov/pubmed/26151029

24. **Dicaffeoyloquinic Acid Enriched Fraction Of Cichorium Glandulosm... (PubMed)**
Tong J (2015) Chicory has a major geographical presence in Europe and Asia. Gichorium glandulosum Boiss. Et Huet, a genus of Cichorium, is used for...
https://www.ncbi.nlm.nih.gov/pubmed/26586022

25. **Amerlioration By Chicory Seed Extract Of Diabetes And Oleic... (PubMed)**
Ziamajidi N (2013) We evaluated the effects of chicory seed extract on hepatic steatosis caused by elary and late stage diabetes in rats (in vivo) and induced...
https://www.ncbi.nlm.nih.gov/pubmed/23603006

26. **Effects Of Chicory Seed Extract On Glucose Tolerance Test And... (PubMed)**
Ghamarian A (2012) The goal was to evaluate and compare the effects of aqueous extract of the seeds of chicory, Cichorium Intybus L, on glucose...
https://www.ncbi.nlm.nih.gov/pubmed/23352214

27. **Effects Of Chinese Herbal Medicine Shenxiong Yujing Granule On... (PubMed)**
Han H (2012) To establish a rat model of diabetes associated cerebral ischemia due to qi and yin deficiency and blood stasis, and to investigate the effects...
https://www.ncbi.nlm.nih.gov/pubmed/23073198

28. **Antihyperglycemic Effects Of Total Flavonoids From Polygonatum... (PubMed)**
Shu XS (2009) Total flavonoids of Polygonatum adoratum were tested for anti-diabetic activity in streptozotocin induced diabetic mice and alloxan induced...
https://www.ncbi.nlm.nih.gov/pubmed/19454312

29. **Hypoglycemic Effects Of Aqueous Extract Of Rhizoma Polygonati... (PubMed)**
Chen H (2001) Water soluble extract of Rhizoma Polygonati Odorati was studied for its hypoglycemic effect in diabetic mice and rats. Results showed that RPO...
https://www.ncbi.nlm.nih.gov/pubmed/11274822

30. **Hypoglycemic Activity Of Polygonati Rhizoma In Normal And... (PubMed)**
Kato A (2008) The hypoglycemic effect of different does of Polygonati Rhizoma was investigated in both normal and streptozotocin induced diabetic mice...
https://www.ncbi.nlm.nih.gov/pubmed/8312868

31. **4-Hydroxyisoleucine: A Potential New Treatment for Type 2 Diabe... (PubMed)**
Zafar MI (2016) 4-Hydroxyisoleucine is a compound found in Trigonella foenum graecum (fenugreek) seeds, which have been used as part of traditional...
https://www.ncbi.nlm.nih.gov/pubmed/27151154

32. **Prevention Effects And Possible Molecular Mechanism Of Mulberry... (PubMed)**
Liu Y (2016) For centuries, mulberry leaf has been used in traditional Chinese medicine for the treatment of diabetes. This study aims to test the prevention...
https://www.ncbi.nlm.nih.gov/pubmed/27054886

33. **Pharmacodynamic Interaction Of Fenugreek, Insulin And Glimepiri... (PubMed)**
Haritha C (2015) this study was undertaken to assess the pharmacodynamics interaction of fenugreek, insulin and glimepiride on sero-biochemical...
https://www.ncbi.nlm.nih.gov/pubmed/27047152

34. **Effectiveness Of Phytotherpy In Supportive Treatment Of Type 2... (PubMed)**
Koupy D (2015) Fenugreek seeds are known for their characteristic smell of soup seasoning and as an ingredient of Indian curry. Traditionally the seeds are used...
https://www.ncbi.nlm.nih.gov/pubmed/26400229

35. **Effect of Fenugreek Seeds on Serum Metabolic Factors and... (PubMed)**
Rafraf M (2014) This triple blind randomized controlled clinical trial was conducted on 88, Type 2 diabetic patients. Subjects in the fenugreek seed...
https://www.ncbi.nlm.nih.gov/pubmed/26098483

36. **Potential Ocular Protection And Dynamic Observation Of Polygona... (PubMed)**
Wang Y (2016) Ocular complications associated with diabetes mellitus are progressive and becoming one of the most important causes of morbidity...
https://www.ncbi.nlm.nih.gov/pubmed/27510582

37. **Antidiabetic Effect Of Total Saponins From Polygonatum Kingianu... (PubMed)**
Lu JM (2016) Polygonatum kingianum has been used in the prevention and treatment of diabetes, hyperlipidemia and related metabolic syndrome in Asian...
https://www.ncbi.nlm.nih.gov/pubmed/26743227

38. **Effects Of Polygonatum Sibiricum Rhizome Ethanol Extract In High... (PubMed)**
Ko JH (2015) the rhizome of Polygonatum sibiricum Redoute has long been used to treat diabetes associated complications. However, the pharmacological...
https://www.ncbi.nlm.nih.gov/pubmed/25327577

39. **Hypoglycemic Action Of the Rhizomes Of Polygonatum Officinale... (PubMed)**
Kato A (1994) the hypoglycemic effect of the rhizomes of Polygonatum officinale was investigated in both normal and streptozotocin induced diabetic mice...
https://www.ncbi.nlm.nih.gov/pubmed/8073082

40. **Effect Of Mulberry Leaf On Insulin Resistance Via IRS-1/PI3k/Glut-4... (PubMed)**
Cai S (2016) Folium Mori, the leaf of Morus alba, has been used in traditional Chinese medicine for treating diabetes. However, it is unclear which...
https://www.ncbi.nlm.nih.gov/pubmed/27158744

41. **The Effects Of Supplementary Mulberry Leaf Extracts On The Trace... (PubMed)**
Krol E (2016) Mulberry leaves have been used in folk medicine to mitigate the symptoms of diabetes. The mulberry plant contains phenolic compounds that...
https://www.ncbi.nlm.nih.gov/pubmed/27071614

42. **Attenuation Of Endoplasmic Reticulum Stress Mediated Liver... (PubMed)**
Afrin R (2016) Endoplasmic reticulum stress plays a crucial role in the development of insulin resistance and diabetes mellitus. Although...
https://www.ncbi.nlm.nih.gov/pubmed/26916916

43. **Mulberry Extract to Modulate Blood Glucose Responses In... (PubMed)**
Lown M (2015) Worldwide sugar consumption has tripled during the last fifty years. High sugar intake is associated with weight gain and increased...
https://www.ncbi.nlm.nih.gov/pubmed/26511964

44. **Morus Nigra Leaf Extract Improves Glycemic Response And Redox... (PubMed)**
Araujo CM (2015) Diabetes mellitus is a chronic metabolic disorder characterized by hyperglycemia and alterations in the carbohydrate, lipid, and protein...
https://www.ncbi.nlm.nih.gov/pubmed/26294257

45. **A Novel Formula From Mulberry Leaf Ameliorates Diabetic Nephro... (PubMed)**
Zhang Q (2015) Based on the hypoglycemia and hyperlipidemia of mulberry leaf and its extracts, we investigated the effects of a novel formula, Sang Tong Jian...
https://www.ncbi.nlm.nih.gov/pubmed/26242486

46. **Mulberry Leaf Extract Improves Postprandial Glucose Response In... (PubMed)**
Kim JY (2015) This study was a randomized, double blind placebo controlled trial to assess the efficacy of 4 weeks of mulberry leaf extract supplementation for...
https://www.ncbi.nlm.nih.gov/pubmed/25343729

47. **A Polysaccharide Extract Of Mulberry Leaf Ameliorates Hepatic... (PubMed)**
Ren C (2015) Mulberry leaf is a traditional medicine used to treat diabetes in the clinic. The aim of this study was to determine the mechanisms by which...
https://www.ncbi.nlm.nih.gov/pubmed/25316427

48. **Dioscorea Extract Modulates Markers Of Peripheral Neuropathy In... (PubMed)**
Moon E (2014) The purpose of this study was to investigate the therapeutic effects of DA-9801, an optimized extract of Dioscorea species, on diabetic...
https://www.ncbi.nlm.nih.gov/pubmed/25414776

49. **Potent Effects Of The Total Saponins From Dioscorea Nipponica... (PubMed)**
Yu H (2015) The aim of the present paper was to investigate the effects and possible mechanisms of the total saponins from Dioscorea nipponica Makino...
https://www.ncbi.nlm.nih.gov/pubmed/25322985

50. **Diosgenin From Dioscorea Bulbifera: Novel Hit For Treatment Of... (PubMed)**
Ghosh S (2014) Diabetes mellitus is a multifactorial metabolic disease characterized by post prandial hyperglycemia. Amylase and glucosidase...
https://www.ncbi.nlm.nih.gov/pubmed/25216353

51. **Anit-Diabetic Effects Of The Ethanol Extract Of A Functional... (PubMed)**
Cheng Q (2015) Phizoma dioscorea, Lycium barbarum, Prunella vulgaris and hawthorn are well known in both traditional food and folk medicine. Each...
https://www.ncbi.nlm.nih.gov/pubmed/24817112

52. **Beta Cell Regenerating Potential Of Azadirachta Indica (Neem) Extr... (PubMed)**
McCalla G (2015) This study evaluated the ability of 0.8% neem leave extract to treat diabetes mellitus by assessing its effects on blood glucose, insulin levels...
https://www.ncbi.nlm.nih.gov/pubmed/26716795

53. **Screening And Design Of Anti-Diabetic Compounds Sourced From... (PubMed)**
Jalil A (2013) Diabetes Mellitus is affecting people of all age groups worldwide. Many synthetic medicines available for type 2 diabetes mellitus in the market...
https://www.ncbi.nlm.nih.gov/pubmed/24497731

54. **Meliacinolin: A Potent Glucosidase And Amylase Inhibitor Isolated... (PubMed)**
Perez-Gutierrez RM (2012) In India, Azadirachta indica is typically known as 'neem tree' and its leaves has long been used in the ayurvedic medical tradition...
https://www.ncbi.nlm.nih.gov/pubmed/22975503

55. **Therapeutic Potential Of Chinese Herbal Medicines In Alcoholic Liver... (PMC)**
Kuan-Hung Lu (2012) Alcoholic liver disease is a complex chronic disease and is associated with a spectrum of liver injury ranging from steatosis and...
https://www.ncbi.nlm.nih.gov/pmc/articles/PMC3942913/

56. **Protective Effect Of Platycodin D On Liver Injury In Alloxan Induce... (PubMed)**
Chen T (2015) Platycodin D is a major pharmacological constituent of Platycodi Radix with immunomodulatory activity. The present study was designed to...
https://www.ncbi.nlm.nih.gov/pubmed/25887267

57. **Platyconic Acid, A Saponin From Platycodi Radix, Improves Glucos... (PubMed)**
Kwon DY (2012) Previous research demonstrated that the crude saponins of Platycodi radix improved glucose metabolism by enhancing insulin sensitivity...
https://www.ncbi.nlm.nih.gov/pubmed/21847688

58. **Long Term Consumption Of Saponins Derived from Platycodi Radi... (PubMed)**
Kwon DY (2009) Crude saponins derived from Chinese Platycodi radix have been reported to prevent increases in body weight and liver TAG in mice fed a high...
https://www.ncbi.nlm.nih.gov/pubmed/18577298

59. **Clinical Efficacy Of Aconitum Containing Traditional Chinese Medic... (PubMed)**
Feng L (2014) Diabetic peripheral neuropathy is a common chronic complication of diabetes. Routine clinical management uses analgesics to relieve pain in...
https://www.ncbi.nlm.nih.gov/pubmed/24467538

60. **Licochalcone E Has An Anti-diabetic Effect... (PubMed)**
Park HG (2012) Licochalcone E is a retrochalcone isolated from the root of Glycyrrhiza inflate. Retrochalcone compounds evidence a variety of pharmacol...
https://www.ncbi.nlm.nih.gov/pubmed/21840191

61. **In Vivo Anti-Diabetic Activity Of Derivatives Of Isoliquiritigenin... (PubMed)**
Gaur R (2014) Isoliquiritigenin, a chalcone and liquiritigenin, a flavonoid found in licorice roots and several other plants. ISL displays antioxidant, anti-inflammato...
https://www.ncbi.nlm.nih.gov/pubmed/24262065

62. **Antidiabetic Effect Of Schisandrae Chinensis Fructus Involves Inhibi... (PubMed)**
Qu Y (2014) Preclinical Research Schisandrae Chinensis Fructus, the fruit of schisandra chinensis is traditionally used as a tonic and anti-diabetes agent in...
https://www.ncbi.nlm.nih.gov/pubmed/25407144

63. **Protective Effect Of Schisandrae Chinensis Oil On Pancreatic B-Cell... (PubMed)**
An L (2015) Islet cell dysfunction in Type 2 diabetes is primarily attributed to increased apoptosis of pancreatic B-Cells. The aim of the present study was...
https://www.ncbi.nlm.nih.gov/pubmed/25151401

64. **Schizandrin Prevents Damage Of Murine Mesangial Cells Via Block... (PubMed)**
Jeong SI (2012) High glucose is the underlying factor contributing to long term complications of diabetes mellitus. Reactive oxygen species have been...
https://www.ncbi.nlm.nih.gov/pubmed/22138248

65. **The Lignin-Rich Fractions Of Fructus Schisandrae Improve insulin... (PubMed)**
Kwon DY (2011) Fructus Schisanddrae, the fruit of Schisandra chinensis, has been traditionally used as a hypoglycemic agent in Asia and its extracts have been...
https://www.ncbi.nlm.nih.gov/pubmed/21440615

66. **Huang-Lian-Jie-Du-Tang Supplemented with Schisandra chinensis... (PubMed)**
Park S (2009) We investigated to determine what effects, if any, the respective water extracts of Radix scutellariae, Fructus schisandrae chinensis (FSC)...
https://www.ncbi.nlm.nih.gov/pubmed/19897925

67. **Anti-Inflammatory And Anti-Superbacterial Properties Of Sulforap... (PMC)**
Woo Jin Choi (2014) Shepherd's purse, Capsella bursa-pastoris Medik, has been considered a health food for centuries in Asia and is known to contain the...
https://www.ncbi.nlm.nih.gov/pmc/articles/PMC3951821/

68. **Herbal Medicines And Nonalcoholic Fatty Liver Disease... (PMC)**
Hong Yao (2016) Nonalcoholic fatty liver disease, which is characterized by excessive fat accumulation in the liver of patients who consume little or no...
https://www.ncbi.nlm.nih.gov/pmc/articles/PMC4974587/

69. **Treatment Of Rats With Jiangzhi Capsule Improves Liquid Fructose... (PMC)**
Yuanyang Zhao (2015) Jiangzhi Capsule is an Australian listed patented traditional Chinese medicine and has been used for management of lipid...
https://www.ncbi.nlm.nih.gov/pmc/articles/PMC4467629/

70. **Crude Extracts From Lycium Barbarum Suppress SREBP-1c Expressi... (PMC)**
Wang Li (2014) Lycium barbarum polysaccharide is well known in traditional Chinese herbal medicine that, has beneficial effects. Previous study reported...
https://www.ncbi.nlm.nih.gov/pmc/articles/PMC4071778/

71. **Recent Advances In The Herbal Treatment Of Non-Alcoholic Fatty... (PMC)**
Jia Xiao (2013) Non-alcoholic fatty liver disease is one of the leading causes of chronic liver injury across the world. It is strongly related to other pathological...
https://www.ncbi.nlm.nih.gov/pmc/articles/PMC3924972/

72. **A Recipe Composed Of Chinese Herbal Active Components regulates... (PMC)**
Sheng-xi Meng (2016) This study is to investigate the therapeutic effects of the recipe composed of Atractylodes macrocephala polysaccharide, chlorogenic...
https://www.ncbi.nlm.nih.gov/pmc/articles/PMC4812184/

73. **Chinese Medicine Formula Lingguizhugan Decoction Improves Beta... (PMC)**
Tao Liu (2013) Lingguizhugan decoction, a classic traditional Chinese medicine formula, has been used to treat obesity and hyperlipidemia in recent years...
https://www.ncbi.nlm.nih.gov/pmc/articles/PMC3664975/

74. **The Liver And Gallbladder Miracle Cleanse: An All-Natural, At-Home... (Book)**
Mortz A (2007) Most people unknowingly suffer from a dangerous buildup of gallstones in the liver and gallbladder. These stones clog up the body's...
http://a.co/jgMBotn